To Ron, my loving husband; Patty, my best friend; Bobbye, my best nurse; and Mom and Dad, my best parents.

C. R. Hart

To my husband Stuart, who encouraged me, and to my children, Elyssa, Brent, David, and Jeremy, who were patient with me during the writing of this book.

M. K. Grossman

*How to Turn Off Your Body's*
*Fat-Making Machine*

# The
# Insulin-
# Resistance
# Diet

CHERYLE R. HART, M.D.
MARY KAY GROSSMAN, R.D.

CB
CONTEMPORARY BOOKS

**Library of Congress Cataloging-in-Publication Data**

Hart, Cheryle R.
    The insulin-resistance diet : how to turn off your body's fat-making machine /
Cheryle R. Hart and Mary Kay Grossman.
      p.   cm.
    Includes bibliographical references and index.
    ISBN 0-8092-2427-5
    1. Reducing diets.    2. Insulin resistance.    3. Weight loss.
I. Grossman, Mary Kay.    II. Title.
RM222.2 .H256    2001
613.2′5—dc21

                                     00-57053

Cover design by Jenny Locke
Interior design by Rattray Design

Published by Contemporary Books
A division of the McGraw-Hill Companies.
4255 West Touhy Avenue, Lincolnwood (Chicago), Illinois 60712-1975 U.S.A.
Printed in the United States of America
International Standard Book Number: 0-8092-2427-5
01  02  03  04  05  06  MV  16  15  14  13  12  11  10  9  8  7  6  5  4  3  2

# Contents

# Acknowledgments

WE WOULD LIKE to thank the following people, who have helped us make this book a reality.

Ron Grossman, editor, word processor, and proofreader of this book: With your constant support and assistance, we have been able to take our research, ideas, and experience and combine them into a book for all to use.

Bobbye Mallory, our longtime nurse and clinic manager: By the example of your own weight-loss success you gave us inspiration to share our medical ideas with other patients.

Our patients at the Wellness Workshop, our clinic: By your faith in following our eating method to control insulin resistance, you have proved to yourself and to the world that this hidden disease can be defeated. You have enabled us to give hope to millions of others like yourselves for whom nothing else has worked until now.

Our literary agent, Jacqueline Simenauer, and her associate Fran Pardi: Thank you for having the foresight to believe in our concepts and the perseverance to find a publisher for this book.

Judith McCarthy, our editor at Contemporary Books: Thank you for recognizing the importance of insulin resistance and for all of your suggestions that helped us refine our ideas and clarify them for our readers. We appreciate all the work that you put into making our book a reality.

Patty Lund, Cheryle Hart's lifelong friend and supporter: You have always come through when I needed you.

# Introduction

THE INSULIN-RESISTANCE DIET is really not a diet book at all. If dieting to you means depriving yourself of the foods you love, combining boring foods with lots of willpower, or starving yourself when you really need to eat—then you are in for a pleasant surprise. *The Insulin-Resistance Diet* is an eating guide. It allows you to eat all the foods that you like in the proper amounts—through our Link-and-Balance Eating Method—and still lose weight. We know how hard it is to lose weight, or even to keep from gaining it. At our medical clinic we have helped thousands of people lose weight and gain control over their appetites and health since we began administering the program in 1996.

"Carbo-loading" in the 1980s made us fat. "Carbo-depriving" in the 1990s made us unhealthy. Yes, that's right. Since most of the popular diets of the 1990s replaced carbohydrates with more protein and fat, we may have lost weight, but our arteries gained fat. The exciting news that you will learn about in *The Insulin-Resistance Diet* is that not only is carbo-deprivation unhealthy, but it's not necessary for weight loss.

*The Insulin-Resistance Diet* will release you from many ideas that are holding you back from healthy living. We will show you how the medical condition *insulin resistance*, which has been associated primarily with prediabetes, is actually present in as many as three out of four overweight people and is making them fat. You can tell if you are likely to have insulin resistance by taking the self-test in Chapter 2. You can control insulin resistance and lose weight by following the simple eating methods we teach in this book.

Once you lose the weight, don't you wish you knew how to keep it off? After you read *The Insulin-Resistance Diet*, you will know how to prevent that weight from coming back. If you are overwhelmed by the huge number of weight-loss diet books and find them hard to follow or just not for you, read the next few pages to find out why *The Insulin-Resistance Diet* is your key to weight loss and control.

## Why You Need to Read This Book

You need to read this book to find out if insulin resistance is the cause of your frustrating weight-loss challenge.

You also need to read it for these reasons:

- To find out if you have insulin resistance. As many as three out of four overweight people have it and don't even know. Do you have it? We'll help you find out.
- To find out if you have Metabolic Syndrome, a weight problem combined with high blood pressure, abnormal cholesterol, abnormal triglycerides, or abnormal glucose tolerance (Type II diabetes).
- To learn how to link and balance what you eat so that you can defeat the deadly combination involved in Metabolic Syndrome.
- If you want to lose weight in the simplest, most effective way—just by learning our Link-and-Balance Eating Method.
- To learn that combining certain foods can cause weight loss, but eating them separately can actually cause weight gain.
- If you want to eat rice, pasta, potatoes, corn, bread, fruit, and sugary foods, but all the other diets say you can't.
- If you don't know about the two-hour fat window and why it is so critical to your weight loss.

- If you want to know what dopamine and serotonin are and how they really control your willpower and appetite.
- If you think you must eat only low-fat, low-calorie foods in order to lose weight.
- If you think you have to do aerobic exercise to lose weight.
- If you've tried every diet, read every book, and exercised all you know how, but you still can't lose weight.
- If you've tried diet pills, but your weight came back—faster than it came off and more of it.
- If you've found other diet plans too complicated, boring, restrictive, or too hard to follow.
- If you want to find out why you *should* splurge on favorite foods in order to lose weight more successfully.
- If you want to understand how we have solved one of the greatest modern mysteries about the body's fat-making machine—turning it off for good using our Link-and-Balance Eating Method, which has controlled weight-loss problems for thousands of our patients.

The Insulin-Resistance Diet, a medically proven way of eating, will naturally lower high blood pressure, cholesterol, and triglycerides. Type II diabetes will also be significantly improved. This means that you may be able to reduce your need for or get off of blood pressure pills, lipid-lowering medications, and even diabetes pills. You and your doctor will be amazed at your improved lab results and health after you follow the nutritional suggestions of this diet for just a short while.

The Link-and-Balance Eating Method is new, unique, and really simple. It is based on the most recent medical and nutritional knowledge about insulin resistance. As many as 75 percent of overweight Americans have this genetic condition, and yet most of us don't even know about it. Not only does this book tell you about this disease, but it also gives you the solution for it. Throw away your calculators, your food scales, your calorie counters, and your fat-gram books. Our gamelike eating approach is fun to follow. You will immediately start losing weight just after using the basic methods of Step 1 (page 27).

This method will work for you because it has worked for thousands who have been where you are right now. Our patients at the Wellness Workshop have experienced weight loss on the average of six to twelve pounds a month—while never feeling deprived or like they're on a diet. Even better, the Link-and-Balance Eating Method results in long-term weight maintenance and improved health without much effort. This book will help you get yourself into the healthy habit of linking and balancing your food.

# Who We Are

We are Cheryle R. Hart, M.D., the founder and medical director, and Mary Kay Grossman, R.D., the nutrition director of the Wellness Workshop in Spokane, Washington. Since 1996, the Wellness Workshop has helped thousands of women and men to lose unwanted pounds and keep them off.

## *From Cheryle R. Hart, M.D.*

Trained at the Mayo Clinic, I have practiced medicine since 1980. During my previous practice as an obstetrician/gynecologist (Ob/Gyn), I became concerned about how many of my obstetric patients had difficulty losing weight after having their babies. I also noticed that many of my other gynecologic patients continuously gained weight over the years. I consulted a locally renowned registered dietitian, Mary Kay Grossman, regarding the steps my patients could take to control their weight. By guiding my patients with her sound nutritional advice, we were able to help some—but not all—of them control their weight. We knew that there was a missing piece of the puzzle needed to solve the weight-loss problems we were seeing.

Our research led us to a medical field called *bariatrics*. Medical researchers and practitioners in this field specialize in helping people to lose and manage their weight. We attended a national bariatric medical conference and learned about a newly discovered condition that affects millions of people trying to lose weight. This condition is called *insulin resistance* or sometimes is referred to as *Syndrome X*. People affected with it have difficulty losing or even maintaining their weight because of their body's reaction to foods that are high in carbohydrates.

Disappointingly, the speakers at the conference offered few guidelines about how people with insulin resistance should eat, other than to limit carbohydrates. To guide our patients, we researched the many popular books that proposed limited carbohydrate diets. Some were not medically sound, while others were extremely complicated. Most were so restrictive that they would be difficult to follow for very long. We were not willing to recommend any of them to our patients. Even though we had found the reason for our patients' weight problems, no one had the solution to long-term weight control.

So we decided to develop our own plan. It had to be safe, easy to understand, have as few restrictions as possible, and still cause weight loss. In this way it would be a plan that our clients could follow for the rest of their lives. For long-term weight control, this was the most important factor. Insulin resistance is a lifelong condition that does not go away, even when the weight does.

## *From Mary Kay Grossman, R.D.*

Being a registered dietitian, I had a good understanding of how foods worked in the body. This knowledge enabled me to figure out which foods would aggravate insulin resistance and which foods should not. As I continued my research, I discovered that I had the condition of insulin resistance. As I began to experiment with meal plans for myself, I noticed that the right combination of foods produced immediate improvement in my energy level and general health. Surprisingly, I found that I was losing weight. This was amazing since I had been unable to lose this weight for seven years since the birth of my first child—even while following what would be considered a healthy, low-fat diet.

Dr. Cheryle Hart and I began to use this plan for all of our patients at the Wellness Workshop. The results were astounding. Even the most challenged patients found that weight loss was easier than ever before. Everyone agreed that the program was easy to understand and very easy to follow. Every day we hear from more people (often shedding tears of joy), thanking us for helping them to finally lose weight and keep it off.

# How to Erase Your Old Dieting Ideas

**Janice**—*Janice is thirty-five years old and never really had any weight or energy problems until after her two pregnancies. She never lost the extra weight she gained with each baby and noticed decreased energy levels. She works long hours and then comes home to care for her family, rarely having much time to sit down for a meal. She experienced afternoon "blahs" and had to perk herself up with a chocolate snack. She lacked her prepregnancy level of energy in the evening. She even saw her doctor about the increased tiredness. Her examination and laboratory studies were all normal. She was very concerned about her extra weight and joined a commercial weight-loss clinic. She was able to lose weight, though very slowly, but was unable to maintain the weight loss because she felt too restricted. Janice was looking for a weight control answer that didn't involve dieting. She came to the Wellness Workshop, and within one week of starting the Link-and-Balance Eating Method, Janice had increased energy and improved concentration at work. She felt less tired in the evening. After two weeks she had lost six pounds. After three months she had achieved her goal of losing twenty-eight pounds. Now, one year later, she still has maintained her lowered weight with her new eating method.*

It's time to reprogram. The very first step to ensuring success with our method is to eliminate all "dieting rules" that proved unsuccessful in the past. Replace them with updated medical facts about weight loss. Read over the common dieting misconceptions below. If you believe any of them, take a really big black marker and cross them out to delete them from your memory banks. (Of course, if you have borrowed this book, mark them out only in your mind.)

### Common Dieting Misconceptions

1. I need to count calories in order to lose weight.

2. I need to count fat grams in order to lose weight.

3. I should do aerobic types of exercises if I expect to lose weight.

4. The best foods to eat when trying to lose weight are low-fat, high-carbohydrate foods, like plain baked potatoes, bagels, or pasta.

5. I should avoid eating meat because it is high in fat and calories.

6. I need to have a will of steel to keep from indulging my cravings.

7. I'll have to give up foods I love to lose weight.

8. Fat-free foods are better for you if you want to lose weight.

9. I will need to follow a strict daily food plan in order to stay focused and lose weight.

10. I have to eat low-calorie foods all of the time in order to lose weight.

We hope that you made your cross-outs really dark so that you won't remember what was under them. Because every one of these statements is false. Stop trying to follow rules that don't work for you.

Now, you can really start over and start losing weight. By following our Link-and-Balance Eating Method you will learn a whole new way to think about food and fat. We have taken the whole science of weight management, all that is scientifically known at this time, and picked, prodded, kneaded, and *thinned out* what we have found to be the simplest and most effective way to lose weight and reclaim your health. We share it with you in the pages of this book. We are looking forward to hearing about your success with our Link-and-Balance Eating Method. Our contact information is on page 223.

# PART I

# How Insulin Resistance Makes Us Fat

# 1

# How Insulin Affects Fat

**M**any people have come to realize over the past ten years that they must be doing something wrong when it comes to weight loss. Despite cutting down on their fat intake by eating fat-free, low-fat, and light food, they keep getting fatter. Did you know that two out of three Americans are now considered overweight? How did this happen when so many people have cut down so well on their fatty food intake?

At our medical clinic, the Wellness Workshop, we've heard it thousands of times. "Doctor, I've never been able to lose weight. I watch my fat intake. I hardly eat anything. In fact, I eat less than everyone else I know does. And I just keep getting fatter!"

*Marsha—Marsha was one of these unfortunate people. She came to us two years ago, after a lifetime of weight gain and dieting, hopeful but preparing herself for another failure. She was on medication for high blood pressure, her cholesterol was very high, and she had recently been told by her doctor that she was in the beginning stages of diabetes. When we looked at her screening for a condition called insulin resistance, it was clear what the problem was. After we had explained to her about the condition, she suddenly saw the reason for all of her weight-loss woes. Just as we anticipated, she did well on our weight-loss plan. Her cholesterol decreased dramatically, and her high blood pressure improved to the point that her doctor felt she could stop her medication. Two years later and forty-two pounds lighter, Marsha has maintained a healthy weight without medication for blood pressure, cholesterol, or diabetes. You can do it too. But first, there are a few things you need to know about insulin and its role in weight gain.*

There is a complex and important relationship between food, blood sugar, insulin, and fat. Insulin helps the body transform food into energy. It helps to regulate blood sugar levels. It also helps *to store fat.* Insulin is a powerful yet hidden fat-building hormone, which is the answer to why we keep getting fatter on low-fat, high-carbohydrate diets.

# How Insulin Turns on Your Fat Switch

Carbohydrates are your body's main source of energy. Carbohydrates include all sugars and honey, all fruits, and all starchy foods such as bread, cereals, pasta, grains, rice, potatoes, and corn. These may be many of the foods you love. All carbohydrates are broken down during digestion into sugars. Glucose is the simplest sugar and the only one that your body can use for energy. Every one of your body's cells needs glucose to function. In fact, the brain relies mainly on glucose. In order to protect the brain, you must maintain a fairly constant level of blood glucose. A blood test would show this normal level to be 80 to 100 mg/dl.

The hormone insulin is the important regulator of your blood glucose levels. Insulin is a hormone just like estrogen, testosterone, thyroid, or cortisone and is secreted into your bloodstream by the pancreas gland. After you eat, digest, and absorb carbohydrate foods, your blood glucose (blood sugar) level normally rises. The pancreas responds by releasing insulin, which then transports glucose into your body cells where it can be used as energy.

If you have more glucose in your body than your cells need, insulin takes extra blood glucose and transports it into fat storage. Blood sugar then returns to normal. This step is important because having abnormally high levels of blood glucose is called *diabetes* and is very damaging to the body.

So, insulin's main job is to regulate blood glucose, and insulin also signals fat storage. When insulin rises and spikes to regulate high blood sugar levels, then more fat is also being stored. This creates some pros and cons when it comes to insulin levels: not enough insulin to regulate high blood sugar levels would result in diabetes, but high insulin levels on a frequent basis will make you fat.

Figure 1.1 shows the normal ups and downs of blood glucose (sugar) levels after eating high-carbohydrate foods. The figure also shows insulin's reaction. Notice the high insulin spike that occurs in the middle to normalize blood sugar levels. It is during this spike that the body makes and stores fat. Surprisingly, the body makes fat as quickly as two to three hours after eating a high-carbohydrate food.

In seeking the real weight-loss solution, the question we asked was simple: "If high insulin levels make you fat, then would *lower* insulin levels make you thin?" The answer is yes. Keeping insulin levels from spiking is the key to your weight-loss solution and is the basis of our Link-and-Balance Eating Method. This unique method teaches you ways to eat every kind of food, even carbohydrates, while keeping your insulin at fat-losing levels.

*Figure 1.1  Glucose and Insulin Response in a Normal Person*

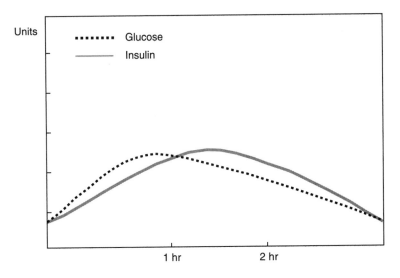

Each unit represents 10 uIU/ml of insulin or 75 mg/dl of blood glucose.

> *High insulin levels mean more body fat, while low insulin levels mean less body fat.*

## Why Some People Gain Weight More Quickly than Others

People have different baseline levels of insulin because of individual genetic makeup. That is, some people just have normally higher levels of insulin than others. People with this condition overreact to carbohydrates with higher-than-normal insulin spikes, so fat storing occurs faster for them. The medical name for this overly high insulin state is called *hyperinsulinemia*. The more common name for this condition is *insulin resistance*.

The more overweight you are, the more resistant to insulin you tend to become. This happens because extra adipose tissue (fat) causes a hormone reaction (a rise in body cortisol) that closes the cells' doors to incoming glucose. The "shunned" glucose has no alternative but to go on to become fat. The good news is that as you lose body fat, the insulin resistance improves, too.

# 2

# Insulin Resistance and Syndrome X

*nsulin resistance* is a condition in which the body does not efficiently use insulin, so your pancreas has to make a lot more insulin to regulate blood glucose. If you have insulin resistance and eat foods high in carbohydrates, up to five times more insulin than normal is needed to bring your blood glucose back down to healthy levels. In fact, some people with insulin resistance produce so much insulin that their blood sugar levels dive way below normal. This low blood sugar condition is called *hypoglycemia*.

## Hypoglycemia

Hypoglycemia causes uncomfortable reactions such as jitteriness, tiredness, mental dullness, headaches, or intense cravings for sugary or starchy foods. Severe hypoglycemia may even be life threatening. People may comment that you are acting grouchy or irritable when your blood sugar level is low. You may not even be aware that you feel so bad until after you eat something and recover. Some people never do associate these symptoms with a real need for body fuel. They only know that they have cravings that will not go away unless they satisfy them. Others simply believe that it is normal to be unproductive after two o'clock in the afternoon unless they follow their daily routine of picking up a cookie at the vending machine.

Many longtime dieters live with feelings of being irritable, tired, and unproductive and enslaved by cravings day in and day out. They assume that if they are trying to lose weight, it is necessary to be hungry much of the time. But all these symptoms of hypoglycemia are not normal and certainly not necessary.

Figure 2.1 shows the glucose and insulin response to eating of someone with insulin resistance resulting in hypoglycemia. Note how high the insulin has to spike to bring down glucose levels. Then note how low the glucose level falls, causing hypoglycemia.

People have varying degrees of severity of this genetically determined condition. If you have insulin resistance, you tend to store most carbohydrates as fat rather than use them as energy. This is probably what has been happening if you've been eating low-fat, low-calorie, yet high-carbohydrate foods and still struggling with your weight. Your frustration likely rose as you got fatter and fatter despite making these sacrifices. This "carbohydrate confusion" is typically seen in people with insulin resistance whose weight loss has been dismal despite their eating nonfat bagels or plain baked potatoes.

*Figure 2.1  Glucose and Insulin Response in a Person
with Insulin Resistance*

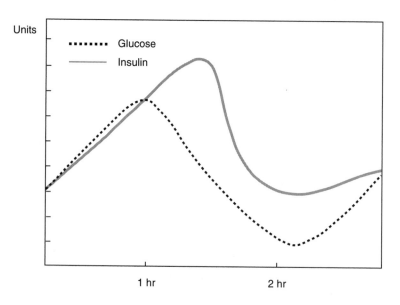

Each unit represents 10 uIU/ml of insulin or 20 mg/dl of blood glucose.

# Syndrome X

In addition to causing obesity, insulin resistance is associated with other serious health problems. In fact, in 1988 Charles Reaven, M.D., of Stanford University, was the first to recognize that a constellation of seemingly unrelated health problems was in fact all caused by a single culprit—insulin. Dr. Reaven termed this condition insulin-resistance syndrome or Metabolic Syndrome. It was known as Syndrome X before insulin was identified as its single cause. Syndrome X involves abnormal blood lipid levels (low HDL cholesterol with high LDL cholesterol and/or high triglycerides), high blood insulin levels, excess body fat (especially around the waist), high blood pressure, increased blood uric acid levels, glucose intolerance (insulin resistance), and blood clotting problems. Having this syndrome places a person at a significantly high risk for having heart attacks, strokes, and diabetes.

Insulin is a powerful hormone. The acronym *CHAOS* can help you remember all the medical problems that excess insulin due to insulin resistance can cause:

C for Coronary artery disease
H for Hypertension
A for Adult-onset diabetes (Type II diabetes)
O for Obesity
S for Stroke

## *Heart Disease*

Too much insulin causes sodium retention, which leads to higher blood pressure. High blood pressure damages blood vessels and results in decreased blood flow to vital organs. The blood vessels of the heart are especially sensitive to this damage. Recent studies now show that even though blood pressure medications satisfactorily control blood pressure, damage is still occurring. The actual risk of heart attacks remains high. This is because the underlying source of the problem, insulin resistance, is still untreated.

Syndrome X also means an increased risk of having a *stroke*, an obstruction of a brain artery. High insulin levels interfere with the clot-dissolving pathway in the bloodstream, so blood clumps more easily and blocks arteries.

Insulin resistance causes changes in blood lipids. These changes can occur regardless of a person's weight. Triglyceride levels go up, bad LDL cholesterol goes up, and good HDL cholesterol goes down. These abnormal changes, called *dyslipidemia*, cause plaque to clog blood vessels and put a person at significant risk for a heart attack or stroke.

Do you know what your *total* cholesterol level is? The guideline of the past was that it should be under 200 mg/dl. We now know that it is really the *ratio* of bad to good cholesterol rather than the total that is most important.

*LDL cholesterol* (low-density lipoprotein) is the "bad" type of cholesterol and should be low. (Remember: you want the one that begins with *L* low.) A level lower than 130 mg/dl is desirable. You are at high risk if your LDL level is over 160 mg/dl.

*HDL cholesterol* (high-density lipoprotein) is the "good" type of cholesterol and should be high. (Remember: you want the one that begins with *H* high). A level higher than 60 mg/dl is best. You are at high risk if your HDL is lower than 35 mg/dl.

*The coronary risk ratio* (LDL/HDL ratio) is the ideal way to identify your true health risk. This ratio should be less than 3.5.

*The cholesterol/HDL ratio* is another ratio used to assess risk. This ratio should be less than 5.0. To determine the ratio, divide your total cholesterol by your HDL. For example, if your total cholesterol is 200 mg/dl and your HDL is 35 mg/dl, the ratio would be 5.7 (200 ÷ 35 = 5.7).

*Triglyceride lipid levels* are considered a separate risk factor for coronary artery disease. The ideal level is 150 mg/dl or lower. If your level is 200 mg/dl or higher, it is important to do something about it (controlling insulin resistance is the key).

To what degree insulin resistance alone is responsible for coronary heart disease is uncertain at this time. An extensive literature review by Ida Chen and Gerald Reaven in 1997 did conclude that insulin resistance plays a key role in the development and clinical course of Type II diabetes as well as hypertension and coronary heart disease.

## Diabetes

Insulin resistance can lead to diabetes later in life. The type of diabetes caused by insulin resistance is called *Type II diabetes*. It has a tendency to run in certain families. One of the theories about how insulin resistance can lead to Type II diabetes is that the insulin supply from the pancreas eventually wears out from all of the challenging years of compensating for high-carbohydrate foods. Without insulin from the pancreas to control it, blood sugar levels rise. Uncontrolled high blood sugar levels (diabetes) cause significant damage to essentially all of the body's organs but especially the heart, blood vessels, liver, eyes, and kidneys. Heart disease and blood vessel damage caused by Type II diabetes are the most common killers of Americans today.

You are particularly at risk for developing Type II diabetes if anyone in your family has had a late-in-life onset of diabetes. Insulin resistance can be considered prediabetes. In fact, studies reveal that diabetes is in the making seven years before it can be clinically diagnosed by high blood sugar levels. This means that if insulin resistance symptoms were recognized and managed early enough, most Type II diabetes could be prevented.

Don't wait until you have the full-blown disease to do something about it. That's like trying to jump on a moving train as it speeds by. Doesn't it make more sense to get on the train while it's stopped at the station? Use the Link-and-Balance Eating Method to prevent the assault of diseases caused by insulin resistance.

In addition to increased risk of heart disease and diabetes, insulin resistance can also cause the following:

> *Premature aging.* Liver spots or "age spots" may show up. Skin tags are those benign, dark- or skin-colored skin flaps that grow on the neck, underarms, chest, and groin. These skin tags are harmless but may be your warning signal of insulin resistance and/or diabetes.

*Increased cancer risk.* Even cancers of the breast, colon, and ovaries have been associated with insulin resistance. Insulin has been shown to promote the growth of malignant cells.

*Gout and kidney stones.* High insulin levels also interfere with the kidneys' ability to clear uric acid from the body. Uric acid is an end product of protein digestion. High levels of uric acid in the blood can result in gout and kidney stones and are also associated with coronary heart disease.

With so many medical problems connected to insulin resistance, it only makes sense to turn our treatment strategies to ways that will defeat it. Winning against insulin resistance allows us to prevent and treat weight problems as well as other serious medical conditions. By lowering insulin resistance we are treating high blood pressure, artery-clogging cholesterol, and heart disease. This wellness approach can prevent these health problems from worsening and may eliminate them completely.

# Why Do So Many People Have Insulin Resistance?

The biological, genetic makeup of modern people very closely resembles that of our primitive Ice Age ancestors. These hunters and gatherers ate mostly meat for their protein and natural grains and berries for their complex carbohydrates. They ate very few refined, simple carbohydrates because they simply weren't available. In fact, despite humans' "modernization" as an evolved species, only five gene changes have been identified since primal humans. Before the modern age, the genetic tendency for insulin resistance was actually a benefit for survival. Those who could easily store fat were more likely to survive a famine. The survivors were more likely to reach adulthood and bear children who would then pass on the insulin resistance gene.

Later, during the agricultural age, humans had easier access to high-carbohydrate foods, such as grains and fruits. Sugary foods are a more recent addition to modern diets. Nowadays, in the Western world you are bombarded with an overabundance of refined carbohydrates that have been marketed to help make your hurried life more convenient. Your body, however, is not equipped to handle the abundance of these types of carbohydrates. Carbohydrates not used as an immediate energy source are turned into stored fat. Along with Americans' increasingly sedentary lifestyle, this explains why, even with the development of low-fat and nonfat food choices, excessive carbohydrates have continued to fatten so many people.

The United States is experiencing an obesity epidemic. One out of every three Americans weighs thirty pounds over his or her ideal weight, and one-half of all Americans are at least 10 percent over their ideal weight. This can be blamed on carbohydrate overload and its consequence: the development of insulin resistance.

## The Insulin-Resistance Roller Coaster

Insulin never has the opportunity to drop down to normal when repeated blasts of glucose from carbohydrates invade the bloodstream. Waves of high insulin cause hypoglycemia. Hypoglycemia makes you crave more carbohydrates. More carbohydrates make glucose . . . glucose needs insulin . . . and the vicious cycle never ends! Remember that insulin takes fat-making along for the ride. Figure 2.2 illustrates this.

Ideally, insulin should gently roll up and down all day long in low hills without having any dramatically high spikes, as in Figure 2.3. This low insulin pattern promotes fat loss.

Lower insulin levels also contribute to improving blood pressure, blood lipids, and other medical problems connected to insulin resistance.

> *Keeping your insulin "calmed down" all day with the powerful Link-and-Balance Eating Method is your weight-loss secret and the key to maintaining your weight and good health.*

*Figure 2.2  Undesirable Insulin and Glucose Response in a Person with Insulin Resistance*

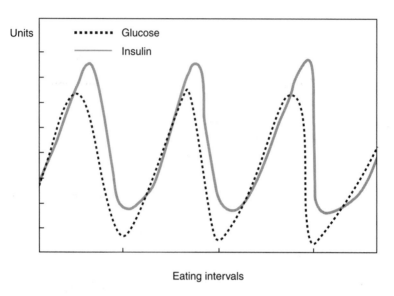

Eating intervals

Each unit represents 10 uIU/ml of insulin or 25 mg/dl of blood glucose. Repeated spikes of insulin and glucose followed by repeated episodes of hypoglycemia are typical in a person with insulin resistance eating a high-carbohydrate diet.

*Figure 2.3  Ideal Insulin and Glucose Response*

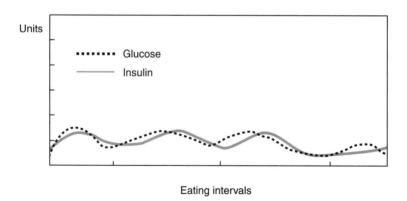

Eating intervals

Each unit represents 10 uIU/ml of insulin or 100 mg/dl of blood glucose.

# Insulin Resistance Self-Test

Do you have insulin resistance? The diagnosis is simple. Read through the self-test list of health conditions and put a check by any items that apply to you.

**Do you have now or have you ever had any of the following?**

- ☑ A family history of diabetes, overweight problems, abnormal cholesterol or triglycerides, heart disease, or stroke
- ☑ Frequent cravings for sweet or salty, crunchy snack food
- ☑ The need to eat often or eat excessive amounts of food
- ☐ A difficult time losing weight even if you exercise or cut back on your food intake
- ☐ A problem with weight gain even when eating small amounts of food
- ☑ Weight gain mostly around your waist
- ☑ Skin tags (small, painless, flappy skin growths) on your neck, chest, breasts, groin area, or underarms
- ☐ A history of irregular menstrual periods, especially skipping months
- ☐ A history of polycystic ovarian disease
- ☑ High triglyceride levels
- ☑ Low HDL cholesterol (the "good" type of cholesterol) levels, that is, lower than 35 mg/dl
- ☑ High LDL cholesterol (the "bad" type of cholesterol) levels, that is, higher than 130 mg/dl
- ☐ High or borderline high blood pressure—even during pregnancy
- ☐ The feeling that you are addicted to carbohydrates
- ☑ The feeling that you have no willpower when it comes to dieting
- ☑ Jitteriness, difficulty thinking, headaches, or nausea that goes away when you eat
- ☐ Hypoglycemia
- ☐ Afternoon fatigue
- ☑ Type II diabetes, borderline diabetes, or abnormal glucose tolerance tests—even just during pregnancy
- ☑ High uric acid or gout

X ☐ History of having a blood clot in your legs, lungs, or brain

X ☐ A doctor telling you that you need to eat less in order to lose weight, yet those close to you are amazed at how little you eat

X ☐ The belief that you are at least thirty pounds overweight

X ☐ A Body Mass Index (BMI) of 30 or higher (see Figure 2.4 to figure your BMI)

X ☐ Native-American, Asian, African-American, or Hispanic ancestry

If you have marked a check beside three or more of these questions, you are likely to have insulin resistance. The more checks you have, the more likely you are to be affected. You are a real target if you have a family history of Type II diabetes, high blood pressure, abnormal lipids, heart attacks, or strokes.

Review your list to see if the items you checked include any one of these:

- High blood pressure
- Low HDL
- High LDL
- High triglycerides
- Overweight by at least thirty pounds
- Body Mass Index of thirty or higher
- Hypoglycemia symptoms
- Abnormal glucose tolerance test
- High uric acid
- Native-American, Hispanic, Asian, or African-American ancestry

If any one of these items applies to you then you are likely to have the full insulin-resistance syndrome or Metabolic Syndrome, and you are at significant risk for developing the health problems we have been talking about.

## Diagnosing Insulin Resistance

You can see your doctor for a laboratory blood test to diagnose insulin resistance if you want to confirm that you are affected or if

### Figure 2.4 Body Mass Index (BMI)

## Height in Inches

| | 60 | 61 | 62 | 63 | 64 | 65 | 66 | 67 | 68 | 69 | 70 | 71 | 72 | 73 | 74 | 75 | 76 |
|---|---|---|---|---|---|---|---|---|---|---|---|---|---|---|---|---|---|
| **100** | 20 | 19 | 18 | 18 | 17 | 17 | 16 | 16 | 15 | 15 | 14 | 14 | 14 | 13 | 13 | 12 | 12 |
| **105** | 21 | 20 | 19 | 19 | 18 | 17 | 17 | 16 | 16 | 16 | 15 | 15 | 14 | 14 | 13 | 13 | 13 |
| **110** | 21 | 21 | 20 | 19 | 19 | 18 | 18 | 17 | 17 | 16 | 16 | 15 | 15 | 15 | 14 | 14 | 13 |
| **115** | 22 | 22 | 21 | 20 | 20 | 19 | 19 | 18 | 17 | 17 | 17 | 16 | 16 | 15 | 15 | 14 | 14 |
| **120** | 23 | 23 | 22 | 21 | 21 | 20 | 19 | 19 | 18 | 18 | 17 | 17 | 16 | 16 | 15 | 15 | 15 |
| **125** | 24 | 24 | 23 | 22 | 21 | 21 | 20 | 20 | 19 | 18 | 18 | 17 | 17 | 16 | 16 | 16 | 15 |
| **130** | 25 | 25 | 24 | 23 | 22 | 22 | 21 | 20 | 20 | 19 | 19 | 18 | 18 | 17 | 17 | 16 | 16 |
| **135** | 26 | 26 | 25 | 24 | 23 | 22 | 22 | 21 | 21 | 20 | 19 | 19 | 18 | 18 | 17 | 17 | 16 |
| **140** | 27 | 26 | 26 | 25 | 24 | 23 | 23 | 22 | 21 | 21 | 20 | 20 | 19 | 18 | 18 | 17 | 17 |
| **145** | 28 | 27 | 27 | 26 | 25 | 24 | 23 | 23 | 22 | 21 | 21 | 20 | 20 | 19 | 19 | 18 | 18 |
| **150** | 29 | 28 | 27 | 27 | 26 | 25 | 24 | 23 | 23 | 22 | 22 | 21 | 20 | 20 | 19 | 19 | 18 |
| **155** | 30 | 29 | 28 | 27 | 27 | 26 | 25 | 24 | 24 | 23 | 22 | 22 | 21 | 20 | 20 | 19 | 19 |
| **160** | 31 | 30 | 29 | 28 | 27 | 27 | 26 | 25 | 24 | 24 | 23 | 22 | 22 | 21 | 21 | 20 | 19 |
| **165** | 32 | 31 | 30 | 29 | 28 | 27 | 27 | 26 | 25 | 24 | 24 | 23 | 22 | 22 | 21 | 21 | 20 |
| **170** | 33 | 32 | 31 | 30 | 29 | 28 | 27 | 27 | 26 | 25 | 24 | 24 | 23 | 22 | 22 | 21 | 21 |
| **175** | 34 | 33 | 32 | 31 | 30 | 29 | 28 | 27 | 27 | 26 | 25 | 24 | 24 | 23 | 22 | 22 | 21 |
| **180** | 35 | 34 | 33 | 32 | 31 | 30 | 29 | 28 | 27 | 27 | 26 | 25 | 24 | 24 | 23 | 22 | 22 |
| **185** | 36 | 35 | 34 | 33 | 32 | 31 | 30 | 29 | 28 | 27 | 27 | 26 | 25 | 24 | 24 | 23 | 23 |
| **190** | 37 | 36 | 35 | 34 | 33 | 32 | 31 | 30 | 29 | 28 | 27 | 26 | 26 | 25 | 24 | 24 | 23 |
| **195** | 38 | 37 | 36 | 35 | 33 | 32 | 31 | 31 | 30 | 29 | 28 | 27 | 26 | 26 | 25 | 24 | 24 |
| **200** | 39 | 38 | 37 | 35 | 34 | 33 | 32 | 31 | 30 | 30 | 29 | 28 | 27 | 26 | 26 | 25 | 24 |
| **205** | 40 | 39 | 37 | 36 | 35 | 34 | 33 | 32 | 31 | 30 | 29 | 29 | 28 | 27 | 26 | 26 | 25 |
| **210** | 41 | 40 | 38 | 37 | 36 | 35 | 34 | 33 | 32 | 31 | 30 | 29 | 28 | 28 | 27 | 26 | 26 |
| **215** | 42 | 41 | 39 | 38 | 37 | 36 | 35 | 34 | 33 | 32 | 31 | 30 | 29 | 28 | 28 | 27 | 26 |
| **220** | 43 | 42 | 40 | 39 | 38 | 37 | 36 | 34 | 33 | 32 | 32 | 31 | 30 | 29 | 28 | 27 | 27 |
| **225** | 44 | 43 | 41 | 40 | 39 | 37 | 36 | 34 | 33 | 32 | 32 | 31 | 30 | 29 | 28 | 27 | 27 |
| **230** | 45 | 43 | 42 | 41 | 39 | 38 | 37 | 36 | 35 | 34 | 33 | 32 | 31 | 30 | 30 | 29 | 28 |
| **235** | 46 | 44 | 43 | 42 | 40 | 39 | 38 | 37 | 36 | 35 | 34 | 33 | 32 | 31 | 30 | 29 | 29 |
| **240** | 47 | 45 | 44 | 43 | 41 | 40 | 39 | 38 | 36 | 35 | 34 | 33 | 33 | 32 | 31 | 30 | 29 |
| **245** | 48 | 46 | 45 | 43 | 42 | 41 | 40 | 38 | 37 | 36 | 35 | 34 | 33 | 32 | 31 | 31 | 30 |
| **250** | 49 | 47 | 46 | 44 | 43 | 42 | 40 | 39 | 38 | 37 | 36 | 36 | 34 | 33 | 32 | 31 | 30 |

*Weight in Pounds*

To use the BMI Chart, intersect your height with your current weight to find your BMI. The shaded BMI (30 or greater) are those at which studies have verified that significant health complications occur due to being overweight, regardless of your current health status.

*Source: Adapted from the* Clinical Guidelines on the Identification, Evaluation, and Treatment of Overweight and Obesity in Adults *by the National Heart, Lung, and Blood Institute (NIH Publication No. 98-4083, page 171, September 1998)*

the self-test results are unclear. Initially your doctor can use a simple fasting glucose level as a guide. This is a blood test that measures your glucose level after you've been fasting for several hours. If this blood sugar level is slightly higher than normal (normal glucose 80 to 100 mg/dl) but not in the diabetic range, you are said to have impaired glucose tolerance. This strongly suggests that you have insulin resistance. You can have insulin resistance, however, even with very normal blood glucose levels. A fasting insulin blood level that is higher than 10 uIU/ml is also a flag for insulin resistance.

The most specific test for diagnosis is a three-hour insulin-glucose tolerance test. This laboratory test involves drinking a pre-measured amount of a special sugar beverage (75 grams glucose load). Your blood is drawn at several hourly intervals and your insulin levels are measured at the same time as the glucose levels. People with insulin resistance have normal to low glucose levels and higher than normal insulin levels.

Normal insulin levels would be in these ranges:

- While fasting, an insulin level of 10 uIU/ml or lower
- After one hour, an insulin level of 50 uIU/ml or lower
- After two hours, an insulin level of 30 uIU/ml or lower
- After three hours, an insulin level of 10 uIU/ml or lower

Research done by J. R. Kraft and colleagues in 1975 showed that any single level of insulin higher than normal gives you the diagnosis of insulin resistance. This was confirmed in 1989 by I. Zavaroni and colleagues.

If you have been diagnosed with Type II diabetes, then you have an extreme degree of insulin resistance. By following the Link-and-Balance Eating Method outlined in this book, you will improve your diabetes condition. You will need to monitor your blood sugar levels because your requirements for oral glucose-regulating medications or injected insulin doses will likely decrease. It is important that your physician monitor this with you. You will want to make a slight change in the way that you link and balance to make sure that you do not put extra stress on your kidneys.

Consult your physician before starting this program. This is especially important if you have diabetes, liver disease, or kidney disease. Your physician will need to know the macronutrient percentages that our method uses.

> *This program provides an approximate daily ratio of 45 percent carbohydrate, 30 percent protein, and 25 percent fat.*

# Factors That Make Insulin Resistance Worse

Certain medications can increase the amount of insulin your pancreas secretes. Some of the most common are the thiazide diuretics, like hydrochlorothiazide, and beta-blockers, such as propranolol. These medications are usually prescribed for high blood pressure control. Steroids, like cortisone or prednisone, also increase insulin resistance. Synthetic progesterone-only birth control pills, injections, or implants worsen insulin resistance. There are even medications prescribed for diabetes control and high cholesterol that actually exacerbate insulin resistance. If you are taking these types of medications, talk to your doctor about their role in insulin resistance. Maybe other effective medications could be substituted.

Caffeine, artificial sweeteners, and nicotine can all cause an increase in insulin. So remember that a diet cola or sweetener in your coffee, even though it has no calories, sends confusing signals to your body. It will not raise blood glucose levels, but insulin levels will increase. The result often leads to low blood sugar levels and hunger.

High levels of stress can worsen insulin resistance because stress activates our "fight or flight" survival mechanism. This stimulates the production of the stress hormone epinephrine. Epinephrine causes the liver and muscles to change glucose from its reserved state, glycogen, to its active sugar form for energy. This causes the glucose levels in your blood to rise. Insulin rises to control high glucose levels. Increased insulin levels then signal fat storing. This explains why some really stressed people cannot lose unwanted weight despite "doing everything right." Learning relaxation techniques to reduce stress can contribute to fat loss and weight maintenance. Massage, hypnotherapy, meditation, prayer, hydrotherapy, and aromatherapy are just a few of the successful methods. You may want to experiment with several of these to see what works best for you.

## Controlling Insulin Resistance

Unfortunately, since we cannot change our genetic makeup at this time, there is no outright cure for insulin resistance. Successful control of insulin resistance is, however, possible and is simple. Controlling it not only results in weight loss but also helps prevent other health problems. The two key elements for the control of insulin resistance are nutrition and physical activity. The Link-and-Balance Eating Method is the most effective nutritional component. Physical activity can take many forms and is discussed more fully in Chapter 10. There are also some prescription medications and natural remedies that may be helpful for insulin resistance treatment.

Newer **prescription medications** for diabetes work either by limiting the liver's release of stored glucose or by letting more glucose into the cells for energy use. These also show promise for the medical treatment of insulin resistance. Currently these medications include glucophage (Metformin), rosiglitazone maleate (Avandia), and pioglitazone (Actos). Other medications are being developed to help glucose get inside the cells for energy rather than be carried off to fat storage.

**Natural supplements** that may be helpful in controlling glucose or insulin include chromium, magnesium, potassium, vanadium, and garcinia cambogia.

> *Chromium* is believed to stabilize blood glucose. Chromium polynicotinate has been found to be the most potent type of chromium. Chromium has also been used to decrease carbohydrate cravings.
>
> *Magnesium* and *potassium* are often deficient inside the cells of persons with insulin resistance. These may need to be supplemented and prescribed by your weight-loss physician. Do not take these without consulting your physician.
>
> *Vanadium* mimics insulin and is believed to help reduce the actual amount of insulin produced by the body.

*Garcinia cambogia* contains hydroxycitrate acid, which signals the body to store glucose in the liver rather than in the fat stores. This is called *glycogen storage*. Glycogen can be used easily for energy when the blood sugar is low.

Do not self-prescribe these supplements by purchasing them yourself at the health food store. Only pharmaceutical grade products that ensure purity and potency are recommended. You should take these supplements only while under the care of a physician trained in the treatment of insulin resistance. Excessive doses of any of these supplements could be toxic, so talk to your physician about the right dosage for your needs.

**Helen**—*When Helen came to see us, she was despondent. She was forty-five years old and had been battling her weight for most of her life. She even remembered going to a doctor for "diet pills" when she was twelve years old. Her whole family seems to have had some type of overweight problem. Her father had diabetes and died of a heart attack at age fifty-seven. Her mother has high blood pressure besides being overweight. Helen herself had a touch of high blood pressure and was worried about a slowly climbing cholesterol level. Her doctor told her that she needed to lose weight but really didn't offer any helpful advice on how to actually accomplish that miracle. Nobody believed her when she told them that she really didn't eat very much but still couldn't lose weight. Helen was an expert on dieting, having tried just about every program out there and read every book. Out of desperation she resorted to trying unsound and unhealthy gimmicks. She had faithfully cut down on her fatty food intake and was even eating her toast plain and putting nothing on her baked potato. Still the fat wouldn't budge. Even exercising didn't help.*

*Helen was puzzled and discouraged by the lack of weight loss despite her conscientious efforts. Her doctor referred her to our Wellness Workshop. It was obvious to us what her problem had been all along. She fit the typical medical profile that we see over one hundred times a month. Helen has insulin-resistance syndrome.*

*By using our Link-and-Balance Eating Method, Helen has been able to lower her blood pressure and cholesterol, as well as lose weight for the first time ever. Her weight loss and control will be her ongoing project over the next several months and even years. She will be getting physically healthier on our program while she is losing weight. She has found the program easy to follow and has never been more hopeful.*

**Kristi**—*Kristi had never needed to watch her weight until after the birth of her first child. She gained fifty-five pounds during her pregnancy, most of which didn't go away after the birth of her nine-and-a-half-pound bouncing baby boy. Although Kristi exercised and tried to cut down on calories for several months, her weight hardly budged.*

*Kristi decided to try a popular high-protein diet that her best friend had recommended. It sounded like it would be easy. She could have all of the meat that she wanted and unlimited amounts of high-fat foods including bacon, mayonnaise, and regular salad dressing. All she had to do was stay away from carbohydrates. During her first week on the diet she learned that this was not going to be as easy as she had thought. Carbohydrates were in everything—especially the foods she loved. Like her friend, she did lose ten pounds in the first month. But every day became more and more difficult.*

*With Kristi's busy lifestyle, cooking separate meals for herself and her family became unmanageable. Joining the family for a quick dinner out was not enjoyable because it meant eating the hamburger without the bun or the pizza without the crust. Special occasions were no longer special for her. It was not fun to watch everyone else enjoy her son's first birthday cake, so she distracted herself in the kitchen. She found herself sampling forbidden foods as she prepared them or snitching French fries from her husband's fast-food tray.*

*Kristi also began to wonder if this diet was really as good for her as was claimed. How could foods that she knew were healthy, such as whole-grain bread, fruits, and nonfat milk, be bad for her? Were high-fat foods including butter and pork rinds really healthy? The authors of her high-protein, high-fat diet book claimed that the craving for sweets would magically disappear, but she found herself daydreaming about eating chocolate bars almost every day. She couldn't wait until she had lost all of her weight so she could have them again.*

*The second month of the diet was even more difficult than the first. To add to Kristi's misery, her weight had stopped going down.*

*She was depressed and hopeless. She could not stand to look at another piece of beef jerky. When she began to notice that her weight was actually starting to go back up again, that was the last straw. She was willing to stay fat for the rest of her life.*

*Fortunately, another friend of Kristi's was a patient at the Wellness Workshop. She had been through a similar experience before starting at our clinic. She told Kristi how much easier it was to fit our plan into her busy lifestyle. She was pleased that her weight loss was consistent at one to two pounds each week since she started our plan. Kristi decided to give weight loss one last try.*

*Now she is happy that she did. After six months of following our program, she lost all of the weight that she wanted to lose. She plans to keep eating this way for the rest of her life. Now that she knows the key to losing weight and keeping it off without making herself miserable in the process, her life is much happier. She feels confident that she is eating healthfully so she can enjoy eating again and still stay slim.*

Now that you know how insulin surges, or spikes, in the blood led to fat storage and weight gain in Helen, Kristi, and many others with insulin resistance, turn to Part II to learn our way to control insulin levels to lose weight and keep it off. We call this program the Link-and-Balance Eating Method.

# PART II
# The Solution to Insulin Resistance
## *The Link-and-Balance Eating Method*

# 3

# Step 1

## *Link Protein*

tudies have shown us that protein foods do not cause insulin to spike and therefore are ideal foods to eat when managing weight problems. Proteins make up the cornerstone of our linking method. *Consult your physician before starting this program if you have ever been told to limit your protein.*

Eating fat with carbohydrates also delays the rise in insulin, but it will not help with weight loss. This is because fat contains more than twice as many calories as protein and carbohydrate. Another concern is that fatty foods do not trigger feelings of fullness, so you are more apt to overeat. In our experience, patients who eat too much fat just don't lose weight.

> Linking *is the simple method of including a food with protein every time you eat, whether or not you also have a food with fat or carbohydrates.*

Linking works because mixing a protein with other foods counteracts and lowers insulin's reaction to those other foods. Other benefits to eating enough protein have to do with fullness and maintaining muscle.

Eating enough protein helps prevent you from getting hungry again too soon. We now know that protein is an important ingredient needed by the body to make *dopamine,* a chemical messenger in the brain that tells you when you are hungry or full. Your dopamine level also is important in maintaining feelings of well-being. Without adequate protein intake you may not be able to make enough dopamine, and you will feel depressed, lack energy, and have significant food cravings. Cravings for chocolate, caffeine, sweets, and fried or salty foods are symptoms of low dopamine.

Another important reason to include adequate protein in your diet is because muscles are made from protein. As you lose weight some muscle is lost because the body finds it easier to use energy stored in muscle protein than in fat. This lost muscle must be replaced or you will end up with less muscle than when you started losing weight. The amount of muscle you have determines how fast your metabolism runs. Less muscle means a slower metabolism, and a slower metabolism means you may regain your weight more quickly.

# High-Protein Foods and How Much to Eat

The following foods are high in protein. You need to have at least one of these every time you eat.

• **Lean meat, fish, poultry, and eggs.** Lean meat choices include flank or sirloin cuts, top round or London broil, and extra-lean ground pork, lamb, or beef. Egg substitutes or egg whites are good high-protein, low-cholesterol choices. You may eat as much of this type of protein as necessary in order to satisfy your hunger. All of your choices should be low-fat.

• **Legumes.** These include dried beans, lentils, peas, and soy products. You may eat as many legumes as necessary to satisfy your hunger.

- **Dairy foods.** Choose milk and milk products that are low-fat or fat-free and have no added sugar, such as cottage cheese and other cheeses. Fat-free or low-fat yogurt with no sugar added is another great protein choice. You may eat as much of these dairy foods as necessary to satisfy your hunger.

- **Nuts and seeds.** These are high in protein but are also high in fat content. You may enjoy four tablespoons of nuts or seeds in a day. We recommend a natural, no-sugar-added brand of peanut butter with the oil poured off. Avoid peanut butters whose labels list sugar as a main ingredient.

Notice that on all but one of these protein choices we say "eat as much as necessary to satisfy your hunger." When you think that you may be satisfied, ask yourself, "Could I stop eating now?" If your answer is "Yes," then you should stop. If your answer is "Yes, but I'd like to have more," you should still stop eating. Just remind yourself that you *can* have more—in two to three hours. If the answer is "Yes, but I'm afraid I'll get hungry before the next meal," then remind yourself that you can satisfy your hunger with a snack before the next meal. Do not gorge yourself or eat until you feel stuffed; reassure yourself that you will not have to go hungry. If you eat to store food for later use, a good portion of it will be stored as fat.

> *Linking works best if you eat protein by itself, before, or with carbohydrates. If this is not possible, then eat some protein as soon after your carbs as you can.*

Here are some examples of linking carbohydrates with protein:

- An apple with a slice of low-fat cheese
- Potatoes with lean meat
- Crackers with low-fat lunch meat or deli meat
- Bread with no-sugar-added peanut butter with the oil poured off

# Sample Linked Meals

You may add coffee, tea, diet sodas, milk, or soy milk to any of the following suggested meals. Protein foods are in **bold** print.

### Breakfasts

An **egg** with toast and vegetable juice

An **omelet** made from eggs or egg substitute with sautéed vegetables and an English muffin with fat-free margarine

No-sugar-added **yogurt** with cereal

Cereal with low-fat or nonfat **milk**

A pancake or waffle with sugar-free syrup and nonfat or low-fat **cottage cheese**

Oatmeal or seven-grain cereal cooked in **milk**

### Lunches

**High-protein light frozen dinners** (15 grams of protein) with **milk** and extra vegetables

Low-fat **lunch meats** spread with low-fat or fat-free **cream cheese** and melon

Low-fat **lunch meats** spread with low-fat condiments on two slices of whole-grain bread

A **meat** and reduced-fat or fat-free **cheese** sandwich and raw vegetables

Grilled **chicken** on a large green salad with fat-free or reduced-fat dressing

A bowl of **chili** or pea, lentil, or **bean soup** with half a grapefruit and vegetable juice

**Vegetable beef soup** with a small amount of potatoes

Vegetable barley soup with lots of **beef** and vegetables

**Lunch meat** and melted reduced-fat **cheese** on half a bagel (preferably whole-wheat, seven-grain, or bran) and a large green salad

Low-fat **tuna** salad with a green salad and a few pretzels

### Dinners

Lean **meat, fish,** or **poultry** with a potato and lots of
vegetables
**Meat, poultry,** or **tofu** stir-fry with rice or noodles
**Meatballs** and melted reduced-fat **cheese** on pasta (preferably
whole wheat, seven-grain, or bran) and a large green
salad
**Lentil** pilaf with steamed vegetables in fat-free **cheese** sauce
One slice thin-crust pizza, topped with **Canadian bacon** or
**ham** and vegetables, and a green salad with low-fat or
fat-free dressing
Chile rellenos with **refried beans** and Mexican rice
Lean **ham** with **black-eyed peas** and vegetables

### Snack Ideas

Low-fat **cheddar cheese** with a small pear
**Beef jerky** with two large rice cakes
No-sugar-added **peanut butter** on celery sticks
Carrot, celery, and jicama dipped in **ricotta cheese** spread or
low-fat ranch dressing
A sandwich with low-fat **lunch meat** and mustard and/or low-
fat mayonnaise
Low-fat or fat-free **cottage cheese** with 1 cup cantaloupe
**String cheese** with crackers
Sugar-free, low-fat **yogurt**
Nonfat or 1 percent **milk** with a graham cracker
Two tablespoons **nuts** and vegetable juice

# Action Plan for Step 1

You can start burning fat as soon as you start Step 1 by linking. Get
used to linking, and then add on at least one new step of our program every two to three days until you have included all of them.
The more you do, the quicker you will lose weight and the more
permanent your weight loss will be.

For the next three days, write down everything you eat in the space below or in a notebook. Identify the high-protein foods by highlighting or circling them. (You may find the food lists in Chapter 4 to be helpful.) Then study your notes. Are you including some high-protein foods at each meal? What could you change or add to those meals to link carbohydrates with protein?

**Day 1 of Linking**

Dinner 1 gluten free toast, cinna + egg, 2 pieces maple sausage fiber drink 1 cup cooked Kale, carrots, radishes

**Day 2 of Linking**

**Day 3 of Linking**

You should be getting the knack of linking by Day 3. You may notice increased energy because your body is using your food more efficiently. Just by including protein foods with each meal or snack your body is producing less insulin and storing fewer carbohydrates as fat. If you feel that you need more practice with linking, continue writing down everything you eat in a notebook as you move on to Step 2 (page 35).

# 4

## Step 2

### *Balance Protein and Carbohydrates*

Think of a balanced meal as a level seesaw. You want to make food choices that will keep the seesaw in balance *every time you eat* whether it's a meal or snack. (See Figure 4.1.) Don't let it tip to either side.

> Linking *means eating a protein every time you eat.*
> Balance *answers the question, "How much protein do I need to link?"*

## How to Plan Meals Using Link and Balance

Keeping your choices in the correct carbohydrate/protein balance is the key to sustaining a healthy weight and a healthy body.

1. You must balance every one serving of a high-carbohydrate food (circle) with one serving of a high-protein food (square). You may stack the rectangle foods in the center of the balance in any amount.

35

*Figure 4.1  Link-and-Balance Seesaw*

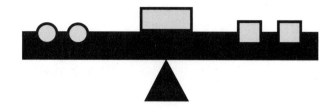

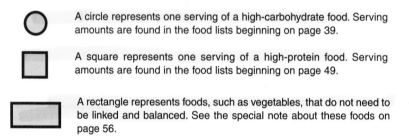

A circle represents one serving of a high-carbohydrate food. Serving amounts are found in the food lists beginning on page 39.

A square represents one serving of a high-protein food. Serving amounts are found in the food lists beginning on page 49.

A rectangle represents foods, such as vegetables, that do not need to be linked and balanced. See the special note about these foods on page 56.

*Figure 4.2  Properly Linked-and-Balanced Seesaw*

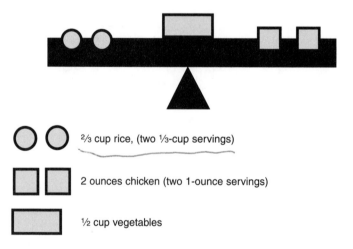

⅔ cup rice, (two ⅓-cup servings)

2 ounces chicken (two 1-ounce servings)

½ cup vegetables

2. Note that Figure 4.1 shows only two circle spaces, allowing for only two high-carbohydrate foods. That is, you are limited to no more than two servings of high-carbohydrate foods at any one meal or snack. This prevents excess carbohydrates from being stored as fat.

*Figure 4.3 Properly Linked-and-Balanced Seesaw*

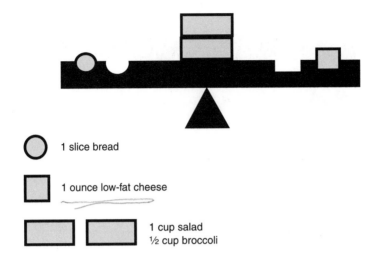

◯  1 slice bread

☐  1 ounce low-fat cheese

▭ ▭  1 cup salad
½ cup broccoli

*Figure 4.4 Properly Linked-and-Balanced Seesaw*

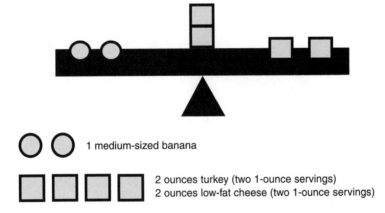

◯ ◯  1 medium-sized banana

☐☐☐☐  2 ounces turkey (two 1-ounce servings)
2 ounces low-fat cheese (two 1-ounce servings)

3. The high-protein foods fit in the two square spaces on the balance. You may also stack them in the middle with the rectangle foods if you desire more. That is, you may have more than two servings of protein if necessary to satisfy your true hunger.

4. Always keep the seesaw in balance with your food choices as in Figures 4.2, 4.3, and 4.4. Do not let it tip to one side or another as in Figures 4.5 and 4.6.

*Figure 4.5   Unbalanced Seesaw*

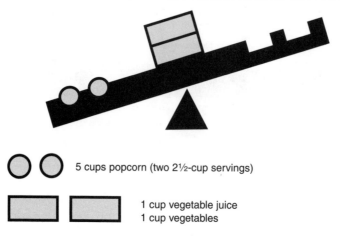

The high-carbohydrate foods in this snack are not linked with protein.

*Figure 4.6   Unbalanced Seesaw*

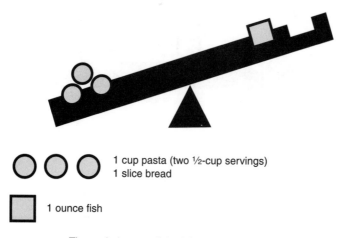

These choices are linked, but they are not balanced.

## Food Lists

The lists that follow are divided into three sections: one for high-carbohydrate foods, another for high-protein foods, and a third for foods high in both carbohydrates and protein. You will find most foods as well as serving sizes, which will help get you started with linking and balancing.

## *High-Carbohydrate Foods*

High-carbohydrate foods include bread and grain products, starchy vegetables, most fruits, and foods that contain large amounts of sugar. These foods cause the greatest increase in blood glucose and insulin and must be limited to just the amount your body needs; otherwise, they will be stored as fat.

You can estimate portions of high-carbohydrate foods without actually measuring. One serving size of high-carbohydrate foods other than the sugary foods is approximately one-half cup, which provides 15 grams of carbohydrates. In order to estimate a half-cup serving of a piece of fruit, for example, try to imagine if it would fit into a half-cup measuring cup. A half-cup serving flattened out is approximately the size and thickness of the palm of a woman's hand or the fingers of a man's hand.

Some fruits, such as raw apples and grapefruit, are not on this list. These fruits are exceptions because they are primarily made up of fructose rather than glucose, so they do not raise your blood glucose and insulin levels. They can be considered rectangle foods when eaten in their raw, unprocessed state. Processing changes their structure, however, so apple or grapefruit *juice* and apple*sauce* are still listed here and must be linked with protein. We will discuss this further in the section on glycemic response on page 72.

## *Fruits*

| Food or Beverage | Serving Size |
| --- | --- |
| Apples, dried, sulfured | 3 slices |
| Apple chips | 9 chips |
| Apple juice | ½ cup |
| Applesauce | |
| sweetened | ⅓ cup |
| unsweetened | ½ cup |
| Apricots | |
| fresh | 4 apricots |
| canned in heavy syrup | ¼ cup (including syrup) |
| canned in juice | ½ cup (including juice) |
| dried halves | 7 halves |

## *Fruits (continued)*

| Food or Beverage | Serving Size |
| --- | --- |
| Apricot nectar, canned | ½ cup |
| Banana | ½ small (8¾-inch length) or ¾ cup |
| Blueberries | |
|    fresh | ¾ cup |
|    frozen, sweetened | ⅓ cup |
| Cantaloupe | ⅓ of a 5-inch-diameter melon |
| Cherries, sweet, fresh | 14 cherries |
| Cranberry juice, light | 1 cup |
| Cranberry juice cocktail | ⅓ cup |
| Cranberry-apple juice | ½ cup |
| Cranberry sauce | 2 tablespoons |
| Dates, whole | 2½ dates |
| Fig, dried | 1 fig |
| Fruit cocktail | |
|    in heavy syrup | ¼ cup |
|    in juice | ½ cup |
| Grapefruit juice | |
|    sweetened | ½ cup |
|    unsweetened | ¾ cup |
| Grapes, green or red, fresh | 17 grapes |
| Grape juice | |
|    sweetened | ⅓ cup |
|    100 percent | ⅓ cup |
|    light | 1 cup |
| Honeydew melon | ⅛ of a 6½-inch-diameter melon |
| Kiwi fruit, fresh | 1½ kiwi fruits |
| Mango, fresh | ½ mango |
| Nectarine, fresh | 1 small (3-inch diameter) or ½ of a large (6-inch diameter) |
| Orange | |
|    fresh | 1 small (3-inch diameter) or ½ of a large (6-inch diameter) |
|    mandarin sections, canned in light syrup | ⅓ cup |
|    juice | ½ cup |

## *Fruits (continued)*

| Food or Beverage | Serving Size |
|---|---|
| Orange-grapefruit juice | ½ cup |
| Papaya, fresh | 1 cup |
| Peach | |
|     fresh | 1 small (3-inch diameter) or ½ of a large (6-inch diameter) |
|     canned in heavy syrup | ¼ cup (including syrup) |
|     canned in juice | ½ cup (including juice) |
|     frozen, sweetened | ¼ cup |
| Pear | |
|     fresh | 1 small (3-inch diameter) or ½ of a large (6-inch diameter) |
|     canned in heavy syrup | ¼ cup (including syrup) |
|     canned in juice | ½ cup (including juice) |
|     dried halves | 1 half |
| Pineapple | |
|     fresh, chunks | ¾ cup |
|     crushed, canned in heavy syrup | ¼ cup (including syrup) |
|     slices, canned in heavy syrup | 1½ slices |
|     crushed, canned in juice | ⅓ cup |
|     slices, canned in juice | 1½ slices |
|     juice, unsweetened | ½ cup |
| Plums | |
|     fresh | 2 medium (2⅛-inch diameter) or 4 small (1½-inch diameter) |
|     canned in heavy syrup | ¼ cup (including syrup) or 2 without syrup |
|     canned in juice | ½ cup (including juice) or 3 without juice |
| Prunes | |
|     dried | 3 prunes |
|     juice | ⅓ cup |
| Raisins | ¾ ounce |

## *Fruits (continued)*

| Food or Beverage | Serving Size |
|---|---|
| Raspberries | |
|     fresh | 1 cup |
|     frozen, sweetened | ¼ cup |
| Strawberries | |
|     fresh | 1½ cups |
|     frozen, sweetened | ¼ cup |
| Tangerine | 1½ tangerines |
| Watermelon, cubed | 1½ cups |

## *Starchy Vegetables*

| Food | Serving Size |
|---|---|
| Corn | ½ cup |
| Potatoes (baked, boiled, microwaved, steamed, scalloped*, au gratin*, French-fried*) | ½ cup |

*High in fat

## *Baked Goods*

| Food | Serving Size |
|---|---|
| Bagel (4-inch diameter) | ⅓ of a bagel |
| Bagel (5½-inch diameter) | ⅕ of a bagel |
| Biscuit* (reduced fat recommended) | 1 (3-inch diameter) |
| Bread crumbs, dry | ¼ cup |
| Bread crumbs, soft | ⅔ cup |
| Bread cubes, soft | 1 cup |

## *Baked Goods (continued)*

| Food | Serving Size |
| --- | --- |
| Bread | |
| Boston brown (3¼-inch diameter) | ⅓-inch slice |
| Cracked wheat, multigrain, oatmeal, white, raisin, or wholewheat (a 1-pound loaf with 18 slices) | 1 slice |
| French, Italian, Vienna, potato, and rye (a 1½-pound loaf with 18 slices) | ⅔ slice |
| French bread baguette (2-inch diameter) | 1¼-inch slice |
| Bread stuffing | ⅓ cup |
| Cake | |
| angel food cake (a 9¾-inch tube cake) | 1/20 of cake |
| frosted double-layer devil's food, white, or yellow cake (8- or 9-inch diameter)* | 1/40 of cake |
| unfrosted cake | 1/25 of cake |
| carrot cake with cream cheese frosting, single layer* | 1 piece (2 inches by 1½ inches) |
| fruitcake | 1/25 of loaf (⅓-inch slice) |
| pound cake (an 8½-inch by 3½-inch by 3¼-inch loaf)* | 1/17 of loaf (½-inch slice) |
| cheesecake (9-inch diameter)* | 1/24 of cake |
| Cookies | |
| brownie, frosted* | 1 (1½-inch by 1¾-inch by 1-inch piece) |
| chocolate chip cookie (2¼-inch diameter)* | ½ cookie |
| fig bar | 1 cookie |
| oatmeal raisin cookie (3-inch diameter)* | ½ cookie |
| peanut butter cookie (3-inch diameter)* | ½ cookie |

## *Baked Goods (continued)*

| Food | Serving Size |
|---|---|
| sugar cookie (2½-inch diameter)* | ½ cookie |
| vanilla wafers | 5 cookies |
| Corn chips* | 1 ounce |
| Crackers | |
| small cheese crackers* | 25 crackers |
| graham crackers | 3 squares |
| matzo | ⅔ matzo |
| melba toast | 4 pieces |
| saltines | 7 crackers |
| Ritz crackers* | 7 crackers |
| Wheat Thins* | 12 crackers |
| Croissant (4½ inches by 4 inches by 1¾ inches)* | ½ croissant |
| Danish pastry* | 1 ounce |
| Doughnuts* | |
| cake type, plain (3¼-inch diameter)* | ½ doughnut |
| yeast leavened, glazed (3¾-inch diameter)* | ½ doughnut |
| English muffin | ½ muffin |
| Muffins, any flavor (2½-inch diameter) | ¾ muffin |
| Pancakes (4-inch diameter) | 2 pancakes |
| Pie (9-inch diameter)* | |
| fruit pie* | 1 wedge 1 inch wide at crust edge |
| cream pie* | 1 wedge 1½ inches wide at crust edge |
| lemon meringue pie* | 1 wedge 1 inch wide at crust edge |
| pecan pie* | 1 wedge 1 inch wide at crust edge |
| pumpkin pie* | 1 wedge 1½ inches wide at crust edge |
| individual snack pies* | ½ pie |
| Pretzels | |
| thin sticks (2¼ inches long) | 63 pretzels |

## Baked Goods (continued)

| Food | Serving Size |
|---|---|
| Dutch twists (2¾ inches by 2⅝ inches) | 1 pretzel |
| thin twists (3¼ inches by 2¼ inches) | 3 pretzels |
| soft pretzels (6 inches by 5 inches) | ⅕ pretzel |
| Rolls and buns | |
| dinner roll (2½-inch diameter) | ¾ roll |
| hot dog bun | ¾ bun |
| hamburger bun | ⅔ bun |
| hard roll (3¾-inch diameter) | ½ roll |
| submarine roll | 3-inch piece |
| Taco shell | 2 shells |
| Toaster pastry* | ½ pastry |
| Tortilla | |
| corn (6-inch diameter) | 1 tortilla |
| flour (8-inch diameter) | 1 tortilla |
| Waffle (7-inch diameter) | ½ waffle |

*High in fat

## Grain Products

| Food | Serving Size |
|---|---|
| Barley, cooked | ⅓ cup |
| Breakfast cereals, cooked | |
| grits or hominy | ½ cup |
| Cream of Wheat | ½ cup |
| Cream of Wheat instant packet, plain | ¾ packet |
| Malt-O-Meal | ½ cup |
| oatmeal | ½ cup |

## *Grain Products (continued)*

| Food | Serving Size |
| --- | --- |
| instant oatmeal, plain | 1 packet |
| instant oatmeal, flavored | ½ packet |
| multigrain cereal | ⅔ cup |
| Breakfast cereals, ready-to-eat | |
| cornflakes | ¾ cup |
| General Mills Cheerios | 1 cup |
| General Mills Golden Grahams | ½ cup |
| General Mills Total | ½ cup |
| General Mills Trix | ⅔ cup |
| General Mills Wheaties | ⅔ cup |
| granola* | ⅕ cup |
| Kellogg's All-Bran | ¼ cup |
| Kellogg's Froot Loops | ⅔ cup |
| Kellogg's Frosted Flakes | ½ cup |
| Kellogg's Product 19 | ½ cup |
| Kellogg's Raisin Bran | ⅓ cup |
| Kellogg's Rice Krispies | ⅔ cup |
| Kellogg's Special K | 1 cup |
| Kellogg's Sugar Smacks | ½ cup |
| Nabisco Shredded Wheat | ½ cup |
| Post Golden Crisp | ½ cup |
| Post Grape Nuts | ¼ cup |
| Post Raisin Bran | ⅓ cup |
| Quaker Oats Cap'n Crunch | ½ cup |
| Quaker Oats Puffed Rice | 1¼ cups |
| Bulgur | ⅓ cup |
| Macaroni | ½ cup |
| Pasta | |
| egg noodles, cooked | ½ cup |
| chow mein, dry | ½ cup |
| spaghetti, fettucine, vermicelli, | |
| and all other pastas | ½ cup |
| Popcorn (Unbuttered is | |
| recommended.) | |
| air-popped or low-fat | 2½ cups |
| popped in oil | 2½ cups |

## Grain Products (continued)

| Food | Serving Size |
| --- | --- |
| caramel-coated | ½ cup |
| Rice, cooked | |
| brown | ⅓ cup |
| white | ⅓ cup |
| instant | ⅓ cup |
| wild | ⅓ cup |
| Wheat germ | |
| raw | ½ cup |
| toasted | ¼ cup |

*High in fat

## Sugary Foods and Sweets

| Food | Serving Size |
| --- | --- |
| Apple butter | 2 tablespoons |
| Caramel | ⅔ ounce |
| Chocolate* | |
| plain | 1 ounce |
| with almonds | 1 ounce |
| with peanuts | 1½ ounces |
| with crisped rice | ¾ ounce |
| chocolate chips | 2½ tablespoons |
| Fondant candies (mints, caramel corn, etc.) | ½ ounce |
| Fudge* | ¾ ounce |
| Gum drops | ⅔ ounce |
| Hard candies, all flavors | ½ ounce |
| Jelly beans | ½ ounce |
| Marshmallows | |
| large | 3 marshmallows |
| small | ⅓ cup |
| Custard, baked with sugar | ½ cup |

## Sugary Foods and Sweets (continued)

| Food | Serving Size |
|---|---|
| Gelatin, regular | ½ cup |
| Honey | 1 tablespoon |
| Jam, jelly, or preserves | 1 tablespoon |
| Popsicle (3-ounce size) | 1 Popsicle |
| Sugar | |
| brown or white | 4 teaspoons |
| powdered | 2½ tablespoons |
| Syrups | |
| corn syrup | 1 tablespoon |
| chocolate, thin | 1⅓ tablespoons |
| chocolate, fudge | 1⅓ tablespoons |
| maple syrup, regular | 1 tablespoon |
| light or reduced-calorie | 2 tablespoons |
| molasses | 1 tablespoon |

*High in fat

## Alcoholic Beverages

| Beverage | Serving Size |
|---|---|
| Beer | 12 ounces |
| Dessert wine | 4 ounces |
| Alcoholic beverages made with fruit or sugary | |
| mixers such as daiquiries or margaritas | 4 ounces |
| Liqueurs | 2 ounces |

Most alcoholic drinks such as wine, whiskey, gin, and vodka are *not* high in carbohydrates and do not need to be considered high-carbohydrate foods. They should be limited to 8 ounces per week, however, in a weight-loss plan.

## Soda Pop

| Beverage | Serving Size |
|---|---|
| All varieties except sugar-free | 4 ounces |

## High-Protein Foods

High-protein foods include most animal products including meats, poultry, fish, eggs, and dairy products. Vegetable proteins such as nuts, dried beans, peas, lentils, and soy products are also included in this group. These foods help to calm the effects of carbohydrates on your blood glucose and insulin levels when they are eaten together.

Don't get confused by the carbohydrates that are found in many high-protein foods such as dairy products and vegetable proteins. These are not used in your body in the same way as other carbohydrates. Thus, these carbohydrates do not need to be considered when linking and balancing.

A one-ounce serving of a high-protein food is approximately the volume of two fingers. A two-ounce serving is approximately the volume of a deck of cards.

## Fish and Shellfish

| Food | Serving Size |
| --- | --- |
| Clams | 1½ ounces |
| Crab meat | 1 ounce |
| Fish sticks* | 1 fish stick |
| Herring, pickled | 1 ounce |
| Oysters | |
|    raw | ⅓ cup |
|    cooked | 1 ounce |
| Lobster meat | 1 ounce |
| Salmon, canned, broiled, baked without added fat, smoked, or fried* | 1 ounce |
| Sardines | |
|    packed in oil* | 1 ounce |
|    packed in mustard, barbecue sauce, etc. | 1 ounce |
| Shrimp, cooked, canned, or fried* | 1 ounce |
| Trout, broiled, baked without added fat, or fried* | 1 ounce |
| Tuna | |
|    water-packed | 1 ounce |
|    packed in oil* | 1 ounce |

## Fish and Shellfish (continued)

| Food | Serving Size |
| --- | --- |
| Whitefish (cod, flounder, sole, haddock, halibut, perch, pollack), steamed, poached, baked without added fat, or fried* | 1 ounce |

*High in fat

## Meat and Poultry

| Food | Serving Size |
| --- | --- |
| **Beef, Pork, and Lamb** | |
| Sirloin, top round, London broil, and flank cuts; braised, roasted, broiled, grilled, or fried* | 1 ounce |
| All other cuts* | 1 ounce |
| Ground beef | |
| less than 10 percent fat | 1 ounce |
| regular*, lean*, or extra-lean* | 1 ounce |
| Heart, liver*, or tongue | 1 ounce |
| Beef jerky | ½ ounce |
| Corned beef* | 1 ounce |
| Chipped beef | 1 ounce |
| | |
| **Poultry** | |
| Chicken or turkey | |
| white meat cooked without skin, broiled, roasted, baked, boiled, or fried* | 1 ounce |
| white meat with skin* | 1 ounce |
| dark meat with or without skin* | 1 ounce |
| chicken or turkey liver* | 1 ounce |
| Duck* or Cornish game hen* | 1 ounce |
| Ostrich or emu | 1 ounce |
| Pheasant cooked without skin | 1 ounce |

## Meat and Poultry (continued)

| Food | Serving Size |
|------|--------------|
| *Processed Meats* | |
| Bologna, beef*, pork*, or turkey* | |
|    regular* | 2 slices |
|    fat-free | 2 slices |
| Braunschweiger* and liverwurst* | 2 ounces |
| Breakfast sausage*, pork* or turkey*, | |
|      links* or patties* | 1 ounce |
| Ham, picnic* or 97 percent lean or leaner | 1 ounce |
| Hot dogs or franks, beef*, pork*, | |
|      chicken*, or turkey* | |
|    regular* | 1½ hot dogs |
|    97 percent lean or leaner | 1½ hot dogs |
| Pepperoni, sliced, regular* or reduced-fat | 17 slices |
| Salami* | |
|    luncheon meat | 2 ounces |
|    dry | 1 ounce |
| Sandwich spread, pork* and beef* | 6 tablespoons |
| Vienna sausages*, pork* and beef* or | |
|      turkey* | 4 sausages |

*High in fat

## Beans, Legumes, Nuts, and Seeds

| Food | Serving Size |
|------|--------------|
| Baked beans | ⅓ cup |
| Black walnuts* | 1 ounce |
| Cashews*, Brazil nuts*, almonds*, | |
|      and English walnuts* | 1½ ounces |
| Chili con carne | ⅓ cup |
| Dried beans (all kinds), lentils, or split peas, | |
|      cooked | ⅓ cup |
| Hummus* | ⅓ cup |

## Beans, Legumes, Nuts, and Seeds (continued)

| Food | Serving Size |
|---|---|
| Macadamia nuts* | 3 ounces |
| Peanut butter* | 2 tablespoons |
| Peanuts* | 1 ounce |
| Pecans* | 3 ounces |
| Pine nuts* | 2 ounces |
| Pistachios, shelled* | 1½ ounces |
| Pumpkin kernels | 1 ounce |
| Refried beans | ⅓ cup |
| Sunflower seeds, shelled* | ¼ cup |
| Tahini (sesame butter)* | 2 tablespoons |

*High in fat

## Dairy Products and Egg Products

| Food or Beverage | Serving Size |
|---|---|
| Buttermilk (low-fat) | 8 fluid ounces |
| Cheese | |
| American, blue, Brie, Camembert, cheddar, Edam, Gorgonzola, Gouda, Gruyère, Monterey Jack, Muenster, Parmesan, Romano, Swiss, regular* or fat-free | 1 ounce |
| mozzarella, part skim or nonfat | 1 ounce |
| Cottage cheese | |
| creamed* | ¼ cup |
| 2%, 1%, or nonfat | ¼ cup |
| dry curd | ⅓ cup |
| Cream cheese, nonfat (Reduced-fat and regular cream cheese do not have adequate protein.) | 3 tablespoons |
| Eggs | |
| whole* | 1 egg |

## Dairy Products and Egg Products (continued)

| Food | Serving Size |
|---|---|
| egg whites | 2 egg whites |
| egg substitutes | ¼ cup |
| Ice cream, frozen yogurt, or ice milk, no sugar added, low-fat, or fat-free (Regular frozen milk desserts that contain sugar must be counted as mixed foods.) | 8 fluid ounces |
| Pudding, sugar-free, made with 1% or nonfat milk (Regular puddings that contain sugar must be counted as mixed foods.) | 1 cup |
| Ricotta cheese | |
| made with whole milk* | ¼ cup |
| made with part-skim milk | ¼ cup |
| Milk (Chocolate milk, eggnog, malted milk, milk shakes, and other flavored milks that contain sugar must be counted as mixed foods unless they are sugar-free.) | |
| nonfat or 1% | 8 fluid ounces |
| 2% or whole* | 8 fluid ounces |
| nonfat dried milk | ⅓ cup (dry) |
| Evaporated milk | |
| whole* | 4 fluid ounces |
| skim | 4 fluid ounces |
| Goat's milk* | 8 fluid ounces |
| Soy milk, unflavored (Flavored soy milks contain sugar and must be counted as mixed foods.) | 8 fluid ounces |
| Yogurt (Yogurt with sugar added must be counted as a mixed food.) | |
| plain | 1 cup |
| flavored, no-sugar-added, lite or light | 1 cup |

*High in fat

## Mixed Foods

The following foods are high in both carbohydrates and protein.

### Mixed Dishes

| Food | Amount | Serving(s) of High-Protein Foods | Serving(s) of High-Carbohydrate Foods |
|---|---|---|---|
| Beef or chicken stew | 1 cup | 2 | 1 |
| Beef or chicken pot pie* | 7 ounces | 3 | 2 |
| Chicken and noodles | 1 cup | 3 | 2 |
| French toast | 1 piece | 1 | 1 |
| Macaroni and cheese, boxed* | 1 cup | 1 | 2 |
| Spaghetti, canned | 1 cup | 1 | 2 |

*High in fat

### Fast Foods

| Food | Amount | Serving(s) of High-Protein Foods | Serving(s) of High-Carbohydrate Foods |
|---|---|---|---|
| Breaded chicken sandwich* | 1 | 3 | 2 |
| Burrito, beef and bean | 1 | 3 | 3 |
| Cheeseburger* | | | |
| regular | 1 | 2 | 2 |
| ¼-pound patty | 1 | 4 | 2 |
| Corn dog* | 1 | 1 | 2 |
| English muffin with egg, cheese, and Canadian bacon | 1 | 2 | 2 |
| Fish sandwich* | 1 | 2 | 2 |

## Fast Foods (continued)

| Food | Amount | Serving(s) of High-Protein Foods | Serving(s) of High-Carbohydrate Foods |
|---|---|---|---|
| Hamburger | | | |
| regular | 1 | 2 | 2 |
| ¼-pound patty* | 1 | 3 | 2 |
| Pizza, plain cheese | ⅛ of 15-inch-round pizza | | |
| thin crust | | 2 | 2 |
| thick crust | | 2 | 4 |
| Roast beef sandwich | 1 | 3 | 2 |
| Taco (without sour cream or guacamole) | 1 | 1 | 1 |

*High in fat

## Snacks (Dairy Foods Containing Sugar)

| Food | Amount | Serving(s) of High-Protein Foods | Serving(s) of High-Carbohydrate Foods |
|---|---|---|---|
| Chocolate milk, eggnog, or malted milk | ½ cup | 1 | 2 |
| Ice cream, regular*, frozen yogurt, or ice milk | ½ cup | ½ | 1 |
| Milk shake* | 1 cup | 1 | 2 |
| Pudding, regular (Low-fat or nonfat is recommended.) | ½ cup | ½ | 1½ |
| Soy milk, flavored | 1 cup | 1 | 1 |

## Snacks (Dairy Foods Containing Sugar, continued)

| Food | Amount | Serving(s) of High-Protein Foods | Serving(s) of High-Carbohydrate Foods |
|---|---|---|---|
| Yogurt, sweetened with corn syrup, honey, or sucrose | 1 cup | 1 | 2 |

*High in fat

## Special Note on Vegetables and Fruits

Vegetables contain both protein and carbohydrates, so they are already balanced. They are mostly made up of water and fiber, so you can use them in large quantities if you desire. You should eat at least three servings per day.

That is, you may eat all vegetables, *except for corn and potatoes*, in unlimited amounts to satisfy hunger. Corn and potatoes are high-carbohydrate foods, and portions must be linked and balanced. They can be found in the lists of high-carbohydrate foods on page 42. Note that *olives and avocados* both have high fat content, and portions must be limited.

You must also consider the method by which the vegetables are prepared. Vegetables that are fried in oil or served with butter or sauces are high in fat and should be eaten sparingly.

Apples, pears, peaches, plums, cherries, and grapefruits do not need to be linked with protein; however, they are not unlimited like vegetables. Eat no more than one half-cup serving every two to three hours. You should eat at least two servings of fruit per day.

# You Can Link and Balance Anything

If you want to eat a food that is not found on our food lists, you simply apply the following formula. This formula automatically helps you to link and balance any food.

## *Balancing Formula*

---

One serving of a carbohydrate is 15 grams.

↓

This is about ½ cup of most high-carbohydrate foods or 1 slice of bread.

You will need to link it with at least 7 grams protein.

↓

Each of these has 7 grams of protein:

1 ounce meat, poultry, or fish

1 slice cheese*

1 piece string cheese*

1 cup milk*

1 cup yogurt*, plain, unsweetened, or sweetened with aspartame or fructose

2 tablespoons peanut butter

3 tablespoons fat-free cream cheese

⅓ cup legumes

1 egg

*Always choose low-fat or nonfat.

---

Remember, you may choose to have less than two servings of a carbohydrate at your meal or snack. However, do *not* exceed two servings (30 grams) at any one time. Always eat enough protein to balance your carbohydrate choices. For example, if you have two servings of high-carbohydrate foods you need two servings (14 grams) of protein.

### Examples of the Balancing Formula

• One slice of toast (15 grams of carbohydrates) links and balances with 1 scrambled egg (7 grams protein).

• Two slices of toast (2 × 15 = 30 grams of carbohydrates) link and balance with 1 cooked egg and 1 cup of low-fat milk (2 × 7 = 14 grams of protein).

• In a sandwich, 2 slices of bread (2 × 15 = 30 grams of carbohydrates) link and balance with at least 2 servings of a high-protein food such as 2 ounces of low-fat or nonfat cheese or 2 ounces of deli meat or tuna (2 × 7 = 14 grams of protein).

• One cup of rice (2 × 15 = 30 grams of carbohydrates) links and balances with at least 2 ounces of chicken (2 × 7 = 14 grams of protein).

• One cup of pasta (2 × 15 = 30 grams of carbohydrates) links and balances with at least 2 ounces of meatballs.

Now try to answer these questions:

*Question:* Does this snack bar have a good balance? The label states that it has 45 grams of carbohydrates and 6 grams of protein.

*Answer:* This snack bar is too high in carbohydrates because it has more than two servings (30 grams) of carbohydrates and not enough protein linking it.

A better balance would be 30 grams of carbohydrates with at least 14 grams protein. Therefore, eating about ¾ of this snack bar and drinking 1 cup of milk with it would make this a properly linked and balanced snack.

*Question:* Can you eat a sandwich made with two pieces of bread and 2 ounces of cheese and add some turkey, too?

*Answer:* Yes, you can.

It's true that the bread and cheese are linked and balanced correctly, but remember, you can always have more protein if you desire. By remembering that protein is always an option, you will never feel hungry or starved.

Just remember, try not to exceed two total fruit, starchy, or sweet carbohydrate servings or a total of 30 grams of carbohydrates in any single meal or snack.

*Question:* Is it OK to eat a snack or meal with a vegetable serving and a protein serving but no carbohydrates?

*Answer:* Yes, it is OK. You must have foods from at least two food groups at each meal. For example, you may choose protein and vegetables, protein and carbohydrates, or all three.

## Food Label Secrets

Use food nutrition labels to stay linked and balanced. One carbohydrate serving is 15 grams and will need to link with at least 7 grams protein. Or two carbohydrate servings is 30 grams and will need to link with at least 14 grams protein. Or, keep this simple label formula in mind:

> Maximum *total carbohydrates of 30 grams links and balances with a* minimum *protein of 14 grams.*

Let's practice link-and-balance label reading. Go to your refrigerator or pantry and take out about four of your favorite foods with labels. Let's read the labels together. First, read how much of the container is a single serving. Now you can properly interpret the numbers we will review. *Stop* reading the calories and fat grams. *Stop* reading the sodium amount unless your doctor has you on a salt-restricted diet for medical reasons. Insulin doesn't care about the calories, and it really doesn't care about the fat grams. We will get more into the recommended amount of dietary fat later in the book. We will always recommend the low-fat choices of all foods, but a certain amount of fat in your diet is essential. We encourage occasional splurging on high-fat delights on special occasions.

Next, read the amount of total carbohydrate grams listed for one serving. The total amount of carbohydrates in one meal or snack portion should not exceed 30 grams. The protein amount to balance this carbohydrate amount should be at least 14 grams. Of course you may only want one carbohydrate serving (15 grams), and so you will only need 7 grams of protein to balance your single serving. Try to stay close to your balance allowance, but you may be off by a few grams of each and still be OK. It is always better to be higher in your proteins than in your carbohydrates.

You may notice that dairy products, legumes, and vegetables do contain some carbohydrates. These carbohydrates do not need to be counted when linking and balancing. The body does not respond to these carbohydrates, which are already linked with protein, in the same way as when you eat high-carbohydrate foods. This is why we consider dairy foods and legumes high-protein foods, too.

You may always exceed two servings of protein if you are hungry. For example, if you feel hungry, drink some low-fat or nonfat milk. Eat some deli meat or cottage cheese. Eat some string cheese. Having protein available to you at any time ensures that you will never feel starved.

## The Two-Hour Fat Window

Eat frequently and think small. Pay attention to what we call the *two-hour fat window.*

*The two-hour fat window is the critical period in which your body decides if carbohydrates are to be used for energy or stored as fat. In order to observe the critical two-hour fat window, limit your total carbohydrates to 30 grams in any two-hour period. This is critical because your body can do only two things with carbohydrates: either use them up as energy or turn them into fat. Your body makes this decision within a two-hour period. Eating more carbohydrates than your body can use for energy during this interval will force your body to turn them into fat. So wait the two hours and then have more carbohydrates if you like. If you are hungry within two hours, you can always have more protein. You can thus continue to enjoy any of your favorite high-carbohydrate foods without overloading and getting fat on them.*

Do eat frequent, small meals. Keep your blood sugar levels more constant by eating at three- to five-hour intervals. Going long periods of time without eating only encourages more fat storage. If you wait too long, your metabolism slows down and fat burning also slows down. Your body shifts into a starvation state. It will hang on to any food eventually eaten by turning most of it into fat. This is the main reason why people who eat only once or twice a day may still have problems losing weight. Their bodies are trying to survive and will not let any fat go for fear of never getting fed again! Studies on long-term weight maintenance show that people who eat *at least five times a day* are the most successful.

## Action Plan for Step 2

Step 2 is the step that will maximize fat burning and minimize fat storage. Here is your action plan for Step 2. Starting now, at each meal or snack, limit your high-carbohydrate foods to no more than two servings. Balance each high-carbohydrate food with at least one high-protein food. Use the food lists to help you. This is linking and balancing.

Record everything that you eat for the next three days. Draw link-and-balance seesaws next to each recording space to make sure you are doing it correctly (see Figure 4.7). Draw your circles, squares, and rectangles to see how your meals balance. Do this for each meal and snack.

**Day 1**

_____

_____

_____

_____

_____

_____

_____

_____

_____

_____

## Day 2

_____

_____

_____

_____

_____

_____

_____

_____

_____

## Day 3

_____

_____

_____

_____

_____

_____

_____

_____

_____

This may take some getting used to, especially if you have a habit of not eating much protein. Carbohydrates are everywhere, but high-protein foods may be hard to find. You will realize this quickly if you rely on vending machines or convenience stores for snacks. Develop some new habits, like bringing high-protein snacks with you. Add more high-protein foods to your routine shopping list. Look for more tips on adding more protein to your diet in Chapter 6.

If for any reason you don't link and balance a meal or snack, don't kick yourself. Use it as a learning experience. Did you feel any different afterward? More sleepy? Less productive? What could you do differently to prevent this in the future? Remember, new behaviors take six to eight weeks to become part of your daily routine. Then, linking and balancing will be more natural for you. A meal won't feel like a meal and a snack won't satisfy you until you have linked and balanced with enough protein. So start developing your new habits now!

> *Step 2: Write down all of your foods as you link and balance them. Visualize the seesaw with every meal and snack.*

*Figure 4.7 Link-and-Balance Seesaw*

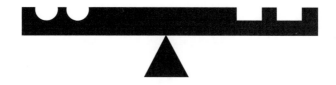

Draw a seesaw such as this for each meal and snack. Insert circles, squares, and rectangles to represent each item of food to make sure each meal or snack balances.

### Simple Balancing Rules

1. Remember to eat from at least two of the food groups.

2. Remember to keep the seesaw balanced. Do not let it tip to one side or another.

Are you feeling more comfortable with linking and balancing now? Keep practicing. Practice makes better—much better! An occasional splurge is helpful and even necessary. Read more about the importance of fulfilling your food interactive needs (foods you can't live without) and appropriate splurging in Chapter 11. For now, try to link and balance most of the time. You will see that even sugary foods such as soda, candy, cake, and cookies can be linked and balanced if you plan carefully and watch the amount.

Don't become too dependent on recording in order to eat properly unless you plan to record *for the rest of your life.* Some people do keep journals or records all of the time, so this may be OK for them. But if you are not one of these people, start to break yourself away from this habit after about six weeks. You may find it helpful to record again for a few days if you get off track, such as during a vacation or after the holidays. Once you are back into the routine you will do fine without keeping a continuous record.

# 5

## Why Link and Balance Works

The Link-and-Balance Eating Method is one that enables you to lose weight without deprivation and avoid the health hazards associated with insulin resistance. Before we introduce the basis behind the Link-and-Balance Eating Method, we want to give you a quick course in nutrition and metabolism. Although the science of nutrition is fairly complicated, there are really just a few things you need to know about nutrition to get a basic understanding of how it applies to weight loss and insulin resistance.

### Nutrition, Weight Loss, and Insulin Resistance

1. The basic nutrients needed by the body are fats, proteins, carbohydrates, water, vitamins, and minerals.

2. Only fats, proteins, and carbohydrates provide energy. These basic nutrients are called *macronutrients*. The energy from food is measured in *kilocalories*. For simplicity, we will continue to refer to kilocalories as just *calories*. Vitamins, minerals, and water do not provide calories and cannot truly give us energy even though they are essential for life.

3. Weight gain will occur if you eat more calories than you use. This is called being in a *positive energy balance*. Weight loss can

happen only if you eat fewer calories than your body uses. In other words, if you have a *negative energy balance.*

4. Fats from plant and animal sources are necessary in small amounts. Your body cannot live without a constant supply of fat. Fats are needed to make hormones and to provide essential fatty acids. However, large amounts of fatty foods make you gain weight because fat is a very concentrated source of calories. Therefore, it is important to eat a low-fat diet, but do not try to eliminate fat from your diet.

5. High-protein foods, which include meat, dairy products, dried beans, nuts, and seeds, are needed for building body tissues, such as muscle. Muscle needs to be made every day. Therefore, you must eat enough rebuilding protein every single day. This is especially true during weight loss, when your body has a tendency to burn up muscle for energy. Extra protein that is not used to make muscle or as energy will be stored as fat.

6. Carbohydrates are needed for energy and are either in simple sugars (such as white sugar or honey) or in complex forms (fruits, breads, pastas, rice, potatoes, corn, and grain). Carbohydrates that are not used as energy will be stored as glycogen or as fat in your body. All carbohydrates (simple or complex) are broken down during digestion into the simple sugars *glucose, fructose*, and *galactose.* Fructose and galactose are eventually changed in the body to glucose. Glucose is the sole sugar that the body's nervous system uses for an energy source. The brain must have a steady source of glucose in order to function properly.

7. It doesn't matter if extra calories come from carbohydrates, proteins, or fats. If you eat more than your body needs, regardless of the calorie source, you will gain weight.

8. Protein and fat can be turned into glucose for energy. But carbohydrates and fats cannot be turned into protein for muscle building. Only a protein can make a muscle. It is for this reason that you must eat adequate amounts of protein daily. Otherwise, *muscle wasting,* or loss of muscle, will occur. The amount of muscle that

your body has sets your *metabolic rate*, the rate at which your body burns calories. The more muscle, the higher your metabolism is. Therefore, muscle loss is very undesirable for weight loss and weight maintenance.

9. Carbohydrates, proteins, and fats in the proper balance are necessary to provide energy, for body tissues and organs, and to keep you at a healthy weight. You should not eliminate any single food group. Even fats, the food group that has gotten the worst rap recently, have a place in a healthy body. Without any fat in your diet you could not make hormones and would become deficient in fat-soluble vitamins and essential fatty acids, all important compounds needed for excellent health.

## How the Science of Nutrition Can Combat Insulin Resistance

Since the identification of insulin resistance, researchers have been scrambling to figure out the best way to handle this condition. The primary goal has been to prevent the onslaught of medical problems associated with it. When we first learned about the condition several years ago, there were very few published guides or articles suggesting any type of dietary recommendations for managing insulin resistance. It was, however, generally recognized that carbohydrate intake must be limited in some way. But which way? Many physicians, realizing that insulin resistance is a result of defective carbohydrate metabolism, began to severely restrict carbohydrate intake to the point of virtually eliminating it from the diet.

This "all or nothing" philosophy banning carbohydrates is not new. In fact, when diabetes was first recognized as a medical condition involving carbohydrate use in the body, physicians recommended eliminating all carbohydrates from the diet. Doing this did keep patients alive a little longer when nothing else was available for diabetes treatment. When insulin injections were discovered as a treatment for diabetes in the 1920s, this dietary restriction still remained the standard of practice, even though there was never any scientific basis to support it. Finally, in the 1970s, studies revealed that diabetics who ate a higher-carbohydrate diet actually improved their blood sugar levels and had fewer cardiovascular complications and therefore lived longer. So now instead of totally eliminating carbohydrates, diabetic specialists actually recommend that 50 to 60 percent of calories in a diabetic diet come from carbohydrates.

In people who are not insulin-resistant, a high-carbohydrate diet does not increase the risk of obesity. In fact, even when overfed carbohydrates, a normal human body will increase its metabolic rate to compensate. Excess carbohydrate intake is first stored as glycogen in the muscle and liver, not in fat tissue. Glycogen is a storage carbohydrate found in all animal proteins and is essential to holding normal blood sugar levels during fasting periods such as sleep and heavy activity. An average adult man is able to store approximately 300 grams of glycogen, enough to sustain energy for about half a day of moderate activity. In this case, very little carbohydrate is turned into fat. This is because activity requires energy, and the body prefers to either burn carbohydrates first for this energy or just store carbohydrates as glycogen. Jean-Marc Schwartz and others confirmed this in their study published in the *Journal of Clinical Investigation* in 1995 but also found that this would not be the case with an insulin-resistant person. They discovered that insulin resistance caused the conversion of carbohydrates to body fat, especially with a very high intake of simple sugars. Clearly, unlimited carbohydrate intake is not desirable for those with insulin resistance, especially the simple forms of carbohydrate. But severely restricting carbohydrates and compensating with just higher protein and/or higher fat in one's diet is also undesirable because the body needs carbohydrates.

When we began working with insulin resistance several years ago, there were no standards of practice, and little scientific knowledge available at that time about diets for this condition. We needed some guidelines to give to our insulin-resistant patients to battle this deadly disease and also achieve safe and healthy weight loss. We studied the recent information that was available. Most information dealing with carbohydrate metabolism had been done in relation to diabetes research. In fact, this research was quite extensive. Because both diseases involve carbohydrate metabolism and are actually just a progression of the same condition, it seemed likely to us that dietary treatment would be similar. Learning from past mistakes, it occurred to us that there was no need to totally eliminate carbohydrates in the diet, as physicians had done when diabetes was first discovered.

## Our Concerns with Very Low Carbohydrate Diets

Many recent popular diet books promote very low carbohydrate intake. We were not anxious to jump on that bandwagon for many reasons.

One great concern of ours about such diets is the fact that many foods that have a high percentage of carbohydrates, such as fruits and whole grains, are also the best sources of antioxidants. *Antioxidants* are the defense agents that help the body prevent disease. Eliminating or severely cutting down on these vital foods would significantly reduce your ability to resist infection, cancer, and aging.

Another concern is that a diet that is low in carbohydrates is usually low in fiber. A low-fiber diet can cause problems with digestion, including constipation and cancers of the digestive tract. A high-fiber diet may actually be protective against development of diabetes. A 1975 study done by H. C. Trowell showed that diabetes deaths dropped during the period of time during and after World War II when fiber intake increased. Many studies have also noted that countries whose citizens have a high fiber intake have low rates of diabetes.

Another interesting group of studies about fiber in the diet involves several ethnic groups who historically have had a high-fiber, high-carbohydrate diet but who now consume diets similar to that of Western cultures, which are very high in carbohydrates and low in fiber. These groups of people have shown a dramatic increase in the incidence of Type II diabetes and insulin resistance. Paul Zimmet, from the Lions-International Diabetes Institute in Melbourne, Australia, has been involved in studies of several island peoples in the South Pacific. He and his colleagues compiled information from many studies in a very interesting report published in 1990. The report illustrates how populations who are genetically inclined to develop insulin resistance and diabetes will do so at an alarming rate when their diet is reduced in fiber and increased in refined carbohydrates even though the carbohydrate intake is relatively unchanged. In all cases, high levels of insulin always occur before diabetes develops. Many of these people also have a dramatic increase in hypertension and heart disease.

W. C. Knowler has been involved in several similar studies about fiber on the Pima Indians of the Southwest United States and confirms Zimmet's results. With their adoption of the typical American diet, one out of every two Pima Indians now develops diabetes. This is among the highest rates of diabetes in the world. Again, it is interesting that the traditional Pima Indian diet has always been high in carbohydrate content; only the fiber intake has decreased. Therefore, it is reasonable to conclude that we should not be so concerned with a high-carbohydrate diet but rather with how much of the carbohydrates are refined and without fiber.

In addition to these health issues, social issues also concern us in considering carbohydrate consumption. We were concerned that a diet that severely limits carbohydrates would be very difficult for anyone to follow for a lifetime. Agriculturally based modern societies are economically and socially dependent on foods that are higher in carbohydrates. You need only look over the party fixings spread across a typical banquet table to see how hard it would be to eliminate carbohydrate foods for a lifetime. Also, humans are born with a preference for sweet foods. Infants will prefer the sweeter milk or sugar water when given a choice. This natural desire for carbohydrates and sweets is difficult, if not impossible, to completely deny.

Another concern with high-protein, high-fat, low-carbohydrate diets is the danger of a medical condition called *ketoacidosis. Ketogenesis*, or the production of ketone bodies, occurs when carbohydrate intake drops to less than about 50 grams per day. Many popular diets recommend ketone production to help with weight loss and appetite control. However, these by-products of fat metabolism can be very damaging to the body and can even result in the dangerous situation ketoacidosis. In this state the body's acid/base balance is disturbed by the acid level of these ketone bodies. The human body is very sensitive to acid/base disturbances, so this can be extremely harmful and even life threatening.

For this reason, it is not advisable for people to follow ketogenic diets unless they are medically supervised by a physician. Fortunately, most people have a very difficult time following these popular ketogenic diets and fudge just enough to prevent them from attaining a ketogenic state. Still, we have seen many others who have been successful in inducing ketogenesis and have ended up in the hospital. The sad part of this story is that it's not necessary. No one has to eat an unhealthy diet to lose weight. We have proven this to be true with thousands of our weight-loss clients over the past several years.

We also have concerns with diets that promote foods with a high fat content. When carbohydrate intake is decreased, an increase in the other macronutrients, protein and fat, is inevitable. Animal protein sources include both fat and cholesterol. High-fat and especially high-cholesterol diets have been shown to contribute to many disease states including heart disease, stroke, and cancer.

Many studies have shown that people who eat diets high in fat are likely to consume more total calories than those who eat diets high in carbohydrates. John E. Blundell from the University of Leeds has participated in several studies regarding fats, carbohydrates, and protein and their effects on human satiety, or how satisfied people feel after eating. A review published by Blundell and his associates in the *American Journal of Clinical Nutrition* in 1994 reported that high-fat foods did not provide satiety signals, which turn off the urge to eat. This then would cause a higher intake of calories. Eating more calories than you need would inevitably cause weight gain. We have found this to be true in many of our patients who have tried to lose weight following popular high-fat, low-carbohydrate diets. The review also showed that foods containing a high amount of carbohydrates do suppress appetite and further notes, "In addition, it is known that when equivalent amounts of energy are given, protein probably exerts the most potent action on satiety of any nutrient." The study concludes that "carbohydrates . . . produce a clear effect on satiety" and that other components such as protein and fiber can modulate and sometimes prolong the satiating action of foods. "Considering these factors, it is possible to design a high-carbohydrate diet that could provide good nutrition with optimum control over appetite and a beneficial effect on body weight."

# The Glycemic Response

In developing our Link-and-Balance Eating Method, we began by limiting only the carbohydrates that were known to have a dramatic effect on raising blood sugar. Blood glucose levels are the stimulating factor for insulin production, and, therefore, preventing high levels of blood glucose is the basis behind maintaining healthy levels of insulin. We were fortunate to have available at the time new research on the glycemic index of foods. We wanted to limit those foods with a *high glycemic response*, or that would raise blood glucose dramatically. There are two recognized ways of looking at the glycemic response. These are the glycemic index and the relative glucose area of foods.

The recently published results of the FAO/WHO Expert Consultation on Carbohydrates in Human Nutrition held in 1997 defined *glycemic index* as "the incremental area under the blood glucose response curve of a 50 gram carbohydrate portion of a test food expressed as a percent of the response to the same amount of carbohydrate from a standard food taken by the same subject." In other words, study subjects are given a standard amount of carbohydrates in a test food, and then their blood sugar is tested for a period of time to see how it is affected. This result is compared to the blood sugar response by the same person to a standard food, usually white bread. This makes it possible to rate foods according to the amount that they affect blood glucose. K. Foster-Powell and J. B. Miller published a compilation of the results of several researchers in 1995. Only a few hundred foods out of the millions of available food choices had been rated at that time, but that was enough to make some valuable conclusions.

Foods with a high glycemic response, such as white and brown sugar, honey, some fruits, and starchy carbohydrates (breads, pastas, cereals, rice, potatoes, and corn) all turn into glucose very quickly and therefore cause a rapid rise in insulin levels. Remember that high insulin spiking induces the body to store fat. Foods that cause a slower glycemic response will not spike insulin levels and are better for people with insulin resistance.

Even though glycemic index research gives us some insight into how foods react in our bodies, there are many inconsistencies in relating this index with the actual response of the body. This makes the glycemic index difficult to use. More recently, several researchers have been interested in determining the relative glucose area (RGA) of foods. This research explains some of the inconsistencies in the glycemic index. Mary C. Gannon, Ph.D., a researcher at the University of Minnesota, has participated in several studies involving different types of carbohydrates and their effect on the relative glucose area as well as serum insulin levels. Dr. Gannon recognized that different types of carbohydrates take different pathways in the body after digestion. Fructose and lactose are both immediately turned into the storage form of sugar, glycogen, in the liver rather than entering the bloodstream as blood glucose. This glycogen pathway gives them much lower glycemic properties than other sugars. So, fruits that are high in fructose do not raise blood sugar significantly and will have a lower glycemic response than fruits that are mostly glucose. Examples of high-fructose fruits are apples and grapefruit. In this same way, milk sugar, or *lactose*, also has a lower glycemic response.

Dr. Gannon also explained that some starchy foods are bound by an outer layer of very complex starches. This encasement increases the time it takes for them to be digested and turned into sugars. These foods, such as beans and other legumes, have a lower glycemic response even though they are relatively high in carbohydrate content.

To simplify our diet recommendations, we chose to limit all fruits, grains, sucrose-containing foods, and those vegetables that do rapidly increase blood sugar. Carrots are not included in our list of limited carbohydrate foods even though they have a high glycemic index. This is because the 50 grams of carbohydrates from carrots required for the test standard far exceed that of a typical portion. Even if a person ate 50 grams of carbohydrates from carrots (that's five cups of carrots), the time it would take to eat the carrots would automatically reduce the glycemic response.

Based on the glycemic response data cited above, we saw no need to limit beans and legumes, dairy products, or vegetables. Even though these foods do contribute a significant amount of carbohydrates to the diet, they have a very small effect on blood glucose and insulin. Eating such foods is a healthy way to include a high proportion of carbohydrates in your diet.

The glycemic index studies also provided us with another important component of our eating method: protein linking. Foods with a high ratio of protein to carbohydrate consistently have lower glycemic values. Dr. Gannon, in conjunction with other researchers, has published several articles showing that eating meals containing both carbohydrates and protein rather than just carbohydrates alone lowers the glycemic response in both normal individuals (nondiabetics) and subjects with Type II diabetes.

At the Wellness Workshop, we began trials with our patients using a diet plan that limited the high-glycemic foods (our foods high in carbohydrates) to the amounts that are generally considered a normal portion. This worked out to be two portions of high-carbohydrate foods at each meal or snack. We recommended patients link protein in a ratio of one serving of protein to each serving of high-carbohydrate food. These recommendations met our goals, which were threefold:

1. Guidelines that are easy to understand and follow

2. Nutritional adequacy and a desirable ratio of macronutrients including a large ratio of carbohydrate, adequate protein, and limited fat

3. The ability to control high glucose responses and resulting insulin reactions leading to fat storage in order to facilitate weight loss and prevent regaining of weight

Our initial trials in 1997 showed such good results that we have changed our recommendations very little since starting the method. Over the past three years, we have treated over three thousand insulin-resistant clients for obesity using this method. In the vast majority of cases, clients are amazed at the results, many finally finding success where they had failed before.

# 6

## Mastering the Link-and-Balance Eating Method

Now that you understand the basic idea of the Link-and-Balance Eating Method, it is time to look at some of the finer points of eating healthfully. Linking and balancing helps your body to use carbohydrates better. But to eat a truly healthy diet, you must also think about other factors. Eating a diet that is high in fat cannot be considered healthy, but not all fat is bad. It would not be healthy to stop eating fruits or to choose only those high-carbohydrate foods that are made from white, unenriched flour and sugar. Eating plenty of vegetables, whole grains, and fruits is very important to good health, as is drinking plenty of water. This chapter will give you some guidelines to complete the picture of a healthy eating plan.

## Protein: The Foundation of the Link-and-Balance Eating Method

As you learn to link and balance, keep in mind that you need to have high-protein foods easily accessible if you are going to successfully link them with more commonly available carbohydrate snacks. Most people starting out on our program either have difficulty eating enough protein or go overboard and eat almost nothing but protein. If you find yourself at either end of the scale, remember that moderation is the key.

To make sure that you get enough protein, keep high-protein snacks handy, add dairy products to your day, and eat eggs and egg substitutes.

# High-Protein Snacks

It's easy to find high-carbohydrate snacks—they're in the vending machine, at the convenience store, at the bakery next door. But high-protein snacks are sometimes hard to find, and if you do find them they are often high-fat options. Get around this by keeping some high-protein foods handy, in your desk drawer at work, in your car, or in your purse or briefcase.

Some good protein snack ideas that you may keep unrefrigerated include the following:

- **Beef or turkey jerky.**

- **Small cans of tuna.**

- **Tuna, fat-free or reduced-fat mayo, and crackers.** At least one national brand packages water-packed tuna with the fixings for tuna salad. Look for it in the tuna section of your grocery store.

- **High-protein snack bars.** Each bar should have at least 7 grams of protein to each 15 grams of carbohydrate. Read labels. Some bars advertised as protein bars are candy bars with a little protein added!

- **Nuts or nut butters.** These products contain more fat than protein, so eat them only occasionally, for a maximum of four tablespoons a day.

- **Instant bean, pea, or lentil soups** in their own cooking cups.

- **Nonfat dry milk.** Add it to coffee, tea, or sugar-free instant cocoa.

- **Shelf-stable microwaveable meals.** These should have at least 15 grams of protein and not more than 35 grams of carbohydrates in each meal.

- **Canned low-fat chili, beans, soups, or stews.** Again, watch the protein to carbohydrate ratio.

The following foods require refrigeration but can be packed in a cooler for lunches or snacks or kept in a refrigerator or freezer if you have one available:

- **Frozen microwaveable meals.** These should have at least 15 grams of protein and not more than 35 grams of carbohydrates.

- **No-sugar-added yogurts.** These are usually labeled "light" or "lite" and are sweetened with aspartame. You may also use plain unsweetened yogurt.

- **Low-fat or nonfat cheeses or cheese sticks.** Regular cheeses other than those made from part-skim milk such as mozzarella have more fat than protein, so eat them only occasionally.

- **Low-fat lunch meats, deli meats, ham, and other processed meats.**

- **No-sugar-added ice cream products.**

- **Low-fat or nonfat cottage cheese.**

- **Hard-cooked eggs.**

## Dairy Products

Even if you dislike milk, use some of these tricks to get the most from the milk that you use in cereal or coffee. Nonfat or 1 percent milk is the best. Other milks contain too much fat.

- Drink "double-strength" milk. Make it by adding nonfat dry milk to fluid milk. Use 1⅓ cups dry milk to each 1 quart of fluid milk or 5⅓ cups dry milk to each 1 gallon of fluid milk.
- Add nonfat dry milk to foods, or cook foods in milk instead of water. For example, use milk when preparing hot cereals, instant coffee, sugar-free cocoa, or tomato soup.
- Add extra nonfat or low-fat cheeses to casseroles, side dishes, and soups. (Keep in mind that boxed macaroni and cheese has very little cheese in it.)
- Have a latte instead of an espresso. Use sugar-free syrups if you like flavorings, because regular syrups have about ninety calories and 22 grams of carbohydrates in each shot.

## Eggs and Egg Substitutes

Fried, poached, soft-cooked, or scrambled eggs are quick to cook in the morning or anytime. We advise you eat no more than three egg yolks each week to keep cholesterol levels low. Use egg substitutes or the egg whites alone once you've met this limit. Even if you're not in the mood for eggs, you can use them to add protein to other foods. Here are some ideas:

- Add beaten eggs to soups and hot cereals when cooking.
- Add diced, hard-cooked eggs to salads or sandwiches.
- Use extra eggs in recipes for casseroles or desserts.

## Protein Essentials Grocery List

Carbohydrates are around every corner. You'll be able to link and balance more successfully if you plan ahead and are "protein prepared." Stash protein foods in your desk, purse, briefcase, car, and workout bag when you leave the house. Remember not to let perishable foods sit too long without refrigeration.

Don't forget these high-protein foods when you shop:

- Skim or reduced-fat milk
- Yogurt (light or no-sugar-added varieties)
- String cheese (nonfat or reduced-fat)
- Nonfat cream cheese
- Cheese (reduced-fat or nonfat)
- Beans
- Beef jerky, turkey jerky
- Cottage cheese (fat-free)
- Peanut butter (natural, with oil poured off the top)
- Lean cuts of meat, fish, and poultry
- Tuna fish packed in water
- Deli meats
- Eggs or egg substitutes
- Sugar-free puddings
- Nonfat, sugar-free ice cream
- Tofu
- Dry-roasted soy nuts

## Get Enough Protein While Limiting Animal Fat

When people think of protein, many of them think of meat. Keep in mind that red meat is just one type of protein. It is a good idea to limit your use of this protein source to a few times each week. Remember that persons with insulin resistance often also have problems with cholesterol and heart disease, so it is wise to eat "heart healthy." Protein sources lower in fat include low-fat dairy products, fish, white poultry meat, lean cuts of pork, soy products, and legumes. Also, use egg whites and cholesterol-free egg substitutes as often as desired. Limit egg yolks, however, to three per week.

Dried beans, peas, lentils (legumes), nuts, and seeds are also high in protein. It is possible to consume adequate protein without eating animal products, but it takes careful planning. The nonmeat protein sources are not complete, meaning that your body cannot use them for muscle building unless they are combined properly with other foods. Books on vegetarianism can give you guidelines. However, unless you use nonanimal sources of protein for a good portion of your protein intake, it is not necessary for you to be concerned with this.

## How Much Protein Is Too Much?

If you eat more calories than your body needs, you will gain weight. It doesn't matter if the calories are protein, carbohydrates, or fat. Start out with a reasonable amount of food. For meat, fish, and poultry, keep to a serving about the size and thickness of the palm of your hand. This should be more than enough to link and balance two servings of high-carbohydrate foods. Enjoy vegetables, low-fat dairy products, and legumes as you desire. If you fill up before you finish, stop eating and save the rest until later. If you are still hungry and you have given your body some time to register that you have eaten (at least twenty minutes from the time you started eating), then take another helping of any food other than the high-carbohydrate foods. An average person requires only about 40 to 70 grams of protein each day (up to 90 grams for a very active athlete). Three to seven servings of high-protein foods, including dairy products, meats, and meat alternatives along with the protein found in some of the high-carbohydrate foods and vegetables should meet this need.

Diets that are made up of mostly protein with little carbohydrates can be dangerous. We do not recommend severely restricting or eliminating carbohydrates from your diet. Dairy products, vegetables, and legumes all contain a fair amount of carbohydrates as well as protein. Even the high-carbohydrate foods (starches, grains, cereals, breads, potatoes, corn, and fruits) should not be eliminated from your diet. This could lead to deficiencies of important vitamins and minerals and could also make you feel hungry or ill because you do not have enough glucose (blood sugar) in your body.

As we have said, the main reason high-protein, very low carbohydrate diets can be dangerous is they may cause your body to make ketones that can be harmful. *Ketones* are produced when your body uses protein instead of carbohydrates for energy. In large amounts, ketones can damage brain cells and cause the minerals in your blood to be unbalanced, which can be life threatening. It is important to give your body adequate carbohydrates to run on throughout the day.

> *Some health conditions require a limit on the amount of protein eaten. The most common is kidney disease. Be sure to consult your physician about your protein food intake if you have such a condition.*

Many of our patients are concerned that protein foods tend to be higher in fats than carbohydrate foods. It is true that a high-fat diet is not healthy and can lead to many diseases, such as heart disease and certain cancers. But remember, do not sacrifice protein for the sake of cutting out fat! In other words, we do not recommend slathering your sandwich with mayonnaise, but we also would not recommend that you forgo some nice lean turkey and have just a tomato sandwich because you are afraid of eating any fat.

## What You Need to Know About Fat in Food

Fat isn't always the bad guy. While eating too much fat can contribute to being overweight, you do need to eat some fat on a daily basis. Your body requires essential fatty acids from fats. A certain amount of the type of fat called *cholesterol* is necessary to produce most of our hormones. Eating too little fat can cause hair loss, skin problems, hormone imbalances, and other health problems.

On the other hand, if you eat large amounts of high-fat foods, you are likely to feel an increased appetite, which can lead to overeating. Studies show that people who eat large amounts of fatty foods eat *one-third more calories* than those who eat less fat.

Experts disagree, however, about exactly how much (or how little) fat is the best amount for a healthy diet. All experts agree that at least 7 percent of your daily calories should come from dietary fats. This is necessary to maintain good health and prevent deficiencies of the essential fatty acids and fat-soluble vitamins. Therefore, a diet that is totally fat-free is not a healthy goal!

Very low fat diets, of less than 20 percent of calories from dietary fat, have been shown to lower cholesterol in some people. A diet this low in fat may not be the best thing, though, if you have insulin resistance, because lowering fat in your diet usually increases the amount of carbohydrates you eat. So for adults with insulin resistance, we recommend a diet containing 20 to 30 percent of calories from dietary fat. This would be the equivalent of 27 to 60 grams of fat per day for most women and 33 to 73 grams for most men. This amount of fat does not excessively increase the amount of carbohydrates you are likely to eat.

A very low fat diet is also never appropriate for children because a critical amount of dietary fat is necessary for brain development during childhood.

Unfortunately, most Americans consume more than 30 percent of calories from dietary fat each day. Don't worry about calculating your daily fat percentage. A simple way to assure that you aren't eating too much fat is to choose foods that are low-fat, meaning that they have less than 3 grams of fat per serving.

If you are like most of our patients, most fat in your diet probably comes from oils and condiments such as butter, margarine, mayonnaise, tartar sauce, and salad dressings. The regular versions of these foods usually contain approximately 5 grams of fat per teaspoon. Try reduced-fat versions of these foods, or simply use less than a teaspoon for each serving.

Some protein foods also can add a significant amount of fat to your diet. However, there are many excellent protein foods that are low-fat, meaning less than 3 grams of fat per serving. Beans and legumes are virtually fat-free. And an eight-ounce glass of 1 percent milk or nonfat milk meets this recommendation. So do one ounce of low-fat or fat-free cheese, one ounce of skinless turkey or chicken breast, one ounce of fish or shellfish, one ounce of pork loin, one ounce of ground beef with less than 10 percent fat, and one ounce of well-trimmed beef top sirloin, top round, or London broil. This does not mean that you must always avoid the higher-fat protein foods that are not low-fat, but you should not make them the staples of your daily intake.

And please do not avoid high-fat proteins and turn to unlinked carbohydrates instead. In other words, if you need to find a snack from the vending machine, pick a protein snack such as peanuts, even if they do have more fat than the peppermint patties or licorice.

Beware when choosing items labeled *reduced-fat*, *low-fat*, or *fat-free*, especially if these are sweet items, desserts, or snack foods such as chips or pretzels. Though low in fat, they are likely to be very high in carbohydrates and very fattening. Food manufacturers know how to trick you into buying their low-fat products by implying that they are healthy.

The 1 or 2 extra grams of carbohydrate in a fat-free mayonnaise compared to a regular mayonnaise are unlikely to make any difference. Don't worry about counting these into your carbohydrate limit.

## *What Types of Fat Are Good for You?*

There is now quite a bit of evidence from medical studies to show that the *types* of fat you eat make a difference. Saturated fats tend to raise cholesterol levels, and eating too much of this kind of fat may worsen insulin resistance. Saturated fats are usually solid at room temperature and include the fats in butter, meats, poultry, milk, egg yolks, coconut oil, and palm oil. This is the kind of fat you want to eat only sparingly.

Polyunsaturated fats and monounsaturated fats, found in liquid vegetable oils, nuts, and seeds, do not have this negative effect, so these are the ones you can have more of. The exception is if they have been *hydrogenated* (hardened) or partially hydrogenated in processing, as in the case of margarines and shortening. This creates harmful products called *transfatty acids*. Transfatty acids can raise the "bad" type of cholesterol (LDL) and lower the "good" cholesterol (HDL).

In addition, the heating and processing of any fat can produce *free radicals*—highly reactive and unstable molecules—which experts strongly believe may cause cancer. Therefore, the best oils are those that are liquid and *cold-pressed* (not heated in processing). Any oil can be cold-pressed. This would be indicated on the front label. Cold-pressed oils are "fragile," tending to spoil easily. Keep them in a dark bottle, refrigerated. Even the normal heating involved in cooking can cause free radicals to form in cold-pressed oils.

Avoid foods that are deep-fried in oil particularly. The high-temperature heating and reheating of the frying oil causes large amounts of free radicals. Using fat-free substitutes such as pan spray when cooking is a great idea. Fat-free margarines have very little saturated fat, hydrogenated fat, or transfatty acids and may be very healthful. There are also some margarines that are labeled "no transfatty acids." Some of these are very good, but be aware because some manufacturers substitute saturated fats such as coconut oil or palm oil, culprits in their own right, comparable to real butter.

Some medical studies now show that there are health benefits from eating higher levels of monounsaturated fats than polyunsaturated or saturated fats. Research has shown that eating a higher proportion of monounsaturated oils, particularly olive oil and canola oil, can prevent high cholesterol levels in the body. Monounsaturated fats do not raise the body's levels of "bad" cholesterol (LDL). Sesame oil, peanuts, almonds, and avocados are also good sources of monounsaturated fats.

Another type of fat, omega-3 fatty acids, has been found to increase the levels of "good" cholesterol (HDL) in the body. Omega-3 fatty acids are an *exception to the rule* when it comes to keeping your dietary fats to 3 grams or less per serving. You can even add up to two tablespoons of these oils each day. This will add as much as two hundred calories to your daily diet but may be helpful especially if your blood studies show low levels of HDL cholesterol. Omega-3 fatty acids can be found in fish oils, flaxseed oil, evening primrose oil, or borage seed oil. You must usually purchase these oils at a health food store. Look for them in the refrigerated section. They are very fragile oils and must be kept cool. Remember that heating oil causes the formation of free radicals. So eat them cold, as in salad dressings or on already-cooked pasta. Some experts recommend using these oils as a daily supplement, especially if you are showing signs of fatty acid deficiency. This includes hair loss, dry hair, dry eyes, dry skin, constipation, and small bumps on the backs of the arms.

## Dietary Fat Action Plan

As we have said, a healthy diet is one that limits your fat to less than 30 percent of your daily intake. This is less than 60 grams per day for most women and less than 73 grams per day for most men. You will be within this guideline if you choose protein foods in the form of lean meats, fish, poultry, and low-fat or fat-free dairy products and make sure the fat you eat in other foods is less than 3 grams per serving. Add up to two tablespoons a day of cold-pressed vegetable oils and/or fish oils.

In addition, gain awareness of the fat content of foods without making it an obsession. Your goal is not to eliminate fat from your daily intake. That would be an impossible diet to maintain and would not be realistic for a lifetime of healthy eating. Begin choosing lower-fat items or limiting the amounts of higher-fat foods to those that will provide 3 grams of fat or less per serving.

Remember, any food that is labeled "low-fat" must contain less than 3 grams of fat per serving by law. Just be careful to eat only the amount listed as one serving. Reduced-fat foods *may contain much more* than 3 grams of fat per serving, so check those labels! And, of course, always remember to link and balance all of your food choices so that eating low-fat foods doesn't give you an overload of carbohydrates.

You may find it helpful to write down what you eat for a few days and identify those foods that are not low-fat by circling or highlighting them.

# Questions About Carbohydrates

We covered a lot of information about carbohydrates in Chapter 4. Once patients get familiar with the program they often have these three important questions.

*Question:* Why do I need carbohydrates at all?

*Answer:* We hear this one most often, particularly in light of all the diets that have made carbohydrates seem like the bad guys. But, in fact, carbohydrates are essential for proper nutrition.

Whole-grain foods such as breads, rice, pastas, cereals, and tortillas are good sources of many minerals (including chromium, which may be helpful for insulin-resistant people). They also supply the vitamins thiamin and niacin and the powerful antioxidant vitamin E. They are important sources of fiber, an essential nutrient for controlling your appetite, as well as preventing constipation. Don't be afraid to eat whole grains and other high-carbohydrate foods every day. Your body needs carbohydrates for energy and to make serotonin, an important brain chemical that tells you when you are no longer hungry. Just be careful not to eat too much of these important foods at one time! Remember to choose the higher-fiber or more complex forms of these foods whenever possible because they provide better nutrition and have lower glycemic indexes, meaning they'll cause less spiking of insulin.

You need fruits, another vitally important group of foods, because they are packed with the antioxidants vitamins C and A. Antioxidants are especially important for people with insulin resistance. We'll discuss more about antioxidants later in this chapter under "Other Foods and Supplements." Fruits also provide folic acid, which you need for building new cells. Not getting enough folic acid causes anemia and can cause birth defects in a developing fetus during pregnancy. Often, when people learn that fruits are high in carbohydrates, they avoid them or limit them too much. Don't be tempted to do this. Include at least two servings of fruits each day. Just be careful not to eat too much fruit or fruit juice at any one time and be sure to link them with protein.

Starchy vegetables such as corn and potatoes also are good sources of many nutrients. You don't have to eliminate them from your diet as long as you keep the portion size down. Just link, balance, and enjoy!

*Question:* Would I be better off never to eat sweets?

*Answer:* Perhaps sugary foods are not the healthiest foods for your physical needs; however, trying to go without any sweets may spell disaster for your emotional health. If you think of some foods as forbidden you may find yourself wanting them even more. There is no reason why you cannot include sugary foods occasionally as long as you link and balance them and keep them as an occasional splurge rather than a routine. Remember that two teaspoons of granulated sugar or honey make up one carbohydrate serving or 15 grams. Always be sure to link your sweets with a protein; for example, fat-free or low-fat milk with a cookie makes a great choice. Learning to splurge safely is an essential skill that you must master in order to achieve long-term weight maintenance. Read more about enjoying sweets and desserts in the section in Chapter 11 about splurging.

There will also be times when you cannot control your food choices, such as at a luncheon meeting or when you are a guest in someone else's home. If you think of yourself as being on a diet, you will feel as though you failed at these times. It is important to accept these events as inevitable and then return to your usual way of eating. This will make it easier to accept this eating method as a lifetime plan rather than a diet. Typically, diets do not work in the long run. Weight loss from dieting is usually followed by weight gain to your previous weight or even higher. Keep in mind that any foods can be part of a healthy diet if used in moderation. So, at your next social gathering, have a small amount of that high-carbohydrate, high-fat food. At the next birthday party, enjoy a small piece of cake and include some protein, like a glass of milk.

*Question:* I crave carbohydrates! What can I do?

*Answer:* It's common for people with insulin resistance to experience cravings for carbohydrates. You may notice that cravings are most likely to occur when you've eaten too many carbohydrates at one time or after you've eaten a food very high in carbohydrates, such as candy. When this happens, your blood sugar rises very quickly, causing your body to produce a sudden high surge of insulin. This large amount of insulin then drives your blood sugar back down rapidly. Your body produces too much insulin compared to the glucose level, and hypoglycemia results.

Your brain relies solely on glucose for thinking and functioning. When low blood glucose occurs, the brain suffers and it demands immediate sugar for relief. This signals an uncontrollable desire or craving for sugary foods. There is no such thing as willpower when your brain is sending strong signals that it needs sugar to rescue it from low glucose levels.

Your satisfying this craving causes another surge of glucose in the blood, which produces another insulin spike. For every glucose surge, an insulin spike follows. Then for every insulin spike, there is a subsequent deep drop in blood glucose. This wild roller-coaster effect continues to cause cravings, which are followed by hypoglycemic reactions. This cycle can repeat *all day long*. Excess fat storing also occurs all day long because of the high insulin production.

Eating adequate amounts of protein and "good" fats seems to be the best remedy for avoiding carbohydrate cravings. Taking chromium supplements may also help control carbohydrate cravings. Researchers have found that many people with insulin resistance and diabetes have chromium deficiencies. Taking chromium to rebuild the body's supply is thought by many to help improve blood glucose levels. Chromium polynicotinate, not chromium picolinate, has been found to be the most potent of these compounds. We have found doses of 200 mcg to 400 mcg three times daily with food to be helpful.

## Tips for Eating More Vegetables and Legumes

Vegetables, legumes, and fruits are good sources of vitamins, minerals, and fiber. And fruits, vegetables, and legumes are the main sources of antioxidants, which are believed to prevent disease, cancer, and premature aging. Unfortunately, eating too many fruits that are high in carbohydrates can lead to fat storage, so you don't want to go overboard on them. Vegetables and legumes have some carbohydrates, but are also high in protein. They provide nutrients without spiking blood sugar, which leads to fat storage. Their high-fiber and low-fat calorie composition will also help to fill you up. So try to eat at least five servings of fruits, vegetables, and legumes every day. Here are some ways:

- Add extra fresh or frozen vegetables to soups, casseroles, and stews.

- Add vegetables to scrambled eggs or omelets.
- Top your salads with vegetables and high-protein beans such as kidney or garbanzo beans.
- Add beans and/or vegetables to rice and pasta dishes.
- Use broccoli and other vegetables as toppings for baked potatoes.
- Don't forget vegetable juices. They are not high in fiber but are packed with other nutrients.
- Include cut raw vegetables as a snack or with your lunch. You may use low-fat or fat-free dip if you wish. Add variety by trying new vegetables you may not normally eat, such as jicama or turnips. You may even discover a new favorite food!
- Make it a habit to include some fruits or vegetables at each meal and perhaps a salad with lunch and dinner.
- If preparation time prevents you from meeting the five-a-day goal, keep ready-to-eat veggies on hand as well as canned and frozen ones. These only take moments to prepare.
- Keep individual cans of vegetable juice on hand in your car or desk drawer to use as a snack or as part of a spur-of-the moment meal.

> *Every once in a while, review what you have eaten throughout the day. If you haven't counted five servings of fruits, vegetables, and legumes, plan ways to work more into your diet in the future. The benefits are worth the effort.*

## Vegetarian Link and Balance

Eating vegetarian meals is a good way to keep fat and cholesterol low. Remember that eating vegetarian does not mean simply leaving the meat out of your spaghetti sauce or leaving the main course item off of your plate and eating only the rice, potatoes, or vegetables. This defeats your purpose, because you will likely eat even more of the high-carbohydrate foods to satisfy your hunger. If these carbohydrates are not linked with protein, your blood sugar and insulin will spike. The insulin spike will cause your body to turn this extra carbohydrate into fat—fat that is very high in cholesterol!

Traditional vegetarian meals include added protein to prevent this. Consider some of these good vegetarian options:

Chili or other Mexican dishes made with beans
Stir-fry meals made with tofu
Middle Eastern dishes made with lentils or garbanzo beans

Can you think of others? These dishes are often served with grain products, usually whole-grain, such as corn bread. Tortillas with beans and rice with stir-fry are common vegetarian combinations. There is an important reason for this. Nonanimal protein sources are not complete. In other words, they do not have all of the protein components you need to make muscle and other body cells. The whole grains have the missing parts. You can also use nuts and seeds, dairy products, or eggs to make a complete protein out of beans, soy products, lentils, and other legumes— but only if you eat them at the same meal. So when you eat nonanimal proteins, be sure to serve them with whole grains or nuts, seeds, dairy products, or eggs. This will link and balance in more than one way!

There are many good books written on vegetarian eating. *Diet for a Small Planet* by Frances Moore Lappé is a very good book on this subject. Please read more about this if you plan to include nonanimal proteins often. Look through the freezer section of your grocery store for new vegetable protein ideas. You'll be surprised at how tasty the prepared foods are now.

# Other Foods and Supplements

Many of our patients have concerns about artificial sweeteners and salt intake. We also receive many questions about nutritional supplements. You'll find our answers in this section.

## Artificial Sweeteners

Sugar has a high carbohydrate content. Therefore, high sugar intake will cause high spikes of insulin. Artificial sweeteners such as saccharin and aspartame do not cause an increase in blood sugar, but they do cause the body to produce small amounts of insulin. This is because the body is fooled into thinking that the blood sugar will go up. If you do use artificial sweeteners, it is important that you *use them with food*, so that the insulin produced will have food to act on. If you drink a diet soda between meals when you are hungry and your blood sugar is low, the extra insulin produced may bring your blood sugar down even lower. (This could explain why some people get headaches after drinking diet sodas.) This reaction can cause you to become excessively hungry or to crave carbohydrates. Avoid this by using artificial sweeteners only when combined with food.

## Salt

Don't worry about salt unless you have been told to do so by your doctor. Limiting salt will not help you truly lose weight. Avoiding salt may keep your body from holding in water, but weight loss from this is temporary. Talk to your doctor if you think you are having trouble with fluid retention.

There is some recent evidence that suggests too much sodium may increase *osteoporosis*, or bone thinning, in postmenopausal women. If you are in this category, it may be wise to avoid foods that are high in sodium such as table salt, soy and Worcestershire sauce, and highly processed foods.

# Vitamin and Calcium Supplements

Let's start our discussion of dietary supplements with calcium. If you do not consistently eat enough dairy products, we strongly recommend you take a calcium supplement to prevent thinning of your bones. People under twenty-four years old need 1,200 to 1,500 milligrams each day. This is approximately equivalent to four to five servings of dairy products, including milk, cheese, yogurt, cottage cheese, or calcium-fortified orange juice. Each serving of these foods contains approximately 300 milligrams of calcium. Women over the age of twenty-five who have not yet reached menopause or who are taking estrogen and men over the age of twenty-five require approximately 1,000 milligrams a day of calcium. This is equal to three servings of high-calcium foods. Postmenopausal women who are not taking estrogen require approximately 1,500 milligrams daily. That's five servings of high-calcium foods.

If you take a multivitamin, it may contain calcium. You can subtract from your daily needs. If you rely on supplements for most of your calcium, you will also need supplemental vitamin D. A multivitamin will meet this need if it contains 100 percent of the recommended daily allowance (RDA) for vitamin D. Otherwise, take a calcium supplement that contains vitamin D.

Determining what brand, type, and amounts of supplements you need can be a daunting task. As with most things, overdoing it can be unhealthy. Using an inferior brand can be a waste of money. Supplements are divided into four quality categories:

1. **Pharmaceutical grade.** This grade meets highest regulatory requirements for purity, dissolution, and absorption and is designated by "USP 23" or says "standardized" or "extract."

2. **Medical grade.** This is a high-grade product. Prenatal vitamins usually fit into this category.

3. **Cosmetic, nutritional grade.** Supplements of this grade are usually sold in health food stores. These often are not tested for purity, dissolution, or absorption and may not have a high concentration of the active ingredient they are labeled as.

4. **Feed or agricultural grade.** Supplements of this grade are used for veterinary purposes. Do not use supplements of this grade.

As for vitamin supplements, most nutritionists agree that the nutrients that you consume in your foods are far superior to those that you can take in a supplement form. This is partly because of the way nutrients interact and partly because we don't yet fully understand all the important elements in food. Certain substances such as phytochemicals, for instance, are present in food but not in supplements. It would therefore be best to consume adequate amounts of various foods to provide all of the essential nutrients. The debatable question is whether or not it is possible to consume all of these foods on a daily basis to achieve optimal health and lose or maintain weight.

The question is further complicated by recent research on the health benefits of taking lots of antioxidants, such as vitamins C and E. Vitamin C is mostly found in fruits, which are also packed with carbohydrates. Vitamin E is found in high-fat foods such as oils. Limiting carbohydrate and fat intake may also, unfortunately, limit your intake of these two nutrients.

If you consistently fail to consume the recommended amounts of foods from all food groups you may become deficient in important nutrients. Limiting the amounts of food that you eat in order to cause weight loss increases the chance that this may happen. If you avoid certain food groups because of allergies or food dislikes, this too increases the risk of nutrient deficiency. It takes effort on your part to make sure that the foods you eat are those that contain high amounts of nutrients. Check to be sure that breads, cereals, rice, and grain foods are whole-grain or fortified. Choose fruit drinks that are 100 percent fruit juice; others do not provide adequate amounts of all vitamins and minerals.

For these reasons we recommend that you take a multiple vitamin supplement when you are trying to lose weight. You may also wish to use a supplement with extra vitamins E and C and take an antioxidant such as grapeseed extract or pinebark extract (pycnogenol) for optimal health benefits. Don't take more than 800 IUs of vitamin E. Taking more than 500 milligrams of vitamin C may not be beneficial, although there is little evidence that it is harmful, especially if you choose a mineral ascorbate form of the vitamin. Nutrient extracts such as grapeseed or pinebark should be standardized to at least 80 percent and taken in amounts of at least 50 milligrams per day. If you take a supplement that is standardized to a lower percent, you may get very little of the actual nutrient, possibly not enough to do any good.

Do try also to get most of your nutrients from the foods that you eat every day. The chart on the following page shows which foods to eat to achieve this.

## High-Nutrient Foods

| Food Group | Sample Foods | Recommended Daily Amount | Main Vitamins and Minerals Provided by These Foods |
|---|---|---|---|
| Dairy foods | Milk, yogurt, buttermilk, cheese, cottage cheese, soy milk | 2 to 5 servings. See text for age-group needs. | Calcium, zinc, vitamin D, and several B vitamins |
| Meat and nonmeat alternatives | Beef, pork, lamb, fish, poultry, eggs, nuts, legumes | A minimum of 3 servings | Iron, zinc, and several B vitamins. A diet low in animal proteins may be deficient in iron and vitamin $B_{12}$. |
| Vegetables | All vegetables | A minimum of 3 servings. Eat a serving of orange or yellow or green leafy vegetables every other day. | Vitamins A and C and several B vitamins |
| Fruit | All fruits | A minimum of 2 servings, one of which should be citrus | Vitamins A and C and folic acid |
| Grains | All whole-grain or enriched bread, cereal, or pasta products | A minimum of 6 servings. But remember to link them with protein and eat no more than 2 servings every 3 hours. | Several B vitamins, iron, and zinc |

# The Wonder of Water

Water suppresses your appetite naturally and helps your body metabolize stored fat. Water is necessary to maximize muscle function. This raises your metabolism. Drinking adequate water is ironically also the best treatment for getting rid of retained excess water. An overweight person needs more water than a thin one because larger people have larger metabolic loads. Since we know that water is the key to fat metabolism, it follows that the overweight person needs more water.

How much water should you drink a day? On the average, a person should drink eight 8-ounce glasses every day. That's about two quarts. The overweight person needs one additional glass for every twenty-five pounds of excess weight. Any noncaffeinated beverages can be counted as fluid to meet your water needs. Caffeine acts as a diuretic and causes fluid loss, so caffeinated beverages cannot be counted as fluids.

## *Action Plan for Drinking More Fluids*

Keep track of the fluids you drink for the next three days. Remember: any liquids that are not caffeinated can be counted as proper fluids. Are you meeting the goals given above? If not, think of ways to include more fluids. Some ideas to help with this include the following:

- Drink herbal teas.
- Drink a full glass of water any time that you brush your teeth, take any vitamins or medication, and eat a meal or snack.
- Have a bottle of water handy when you sit down at your desk to work, watch TV, do physical activity, and drive in your car.
- Keep filtered water, lemon water, or herbal iced tea in your refrigerator.
- Freeze two bottles of water every night—one to take to work and drink as it thaws and one to take in your lunch to keep your food cool and then drink throughout the afternoon.

As a summary of relative amounts and importance of the various categories of foods just presented, we offer our Link-and-Balance Food Pyramid (see Figure 6.1).

This pyramid is like the one shown on the side of cereal boxes in a very important way. As in both pyramids, the base shows the types of foods that we want more of. The closer to the top, the less of those foods we eat. The difference is in the order ranking of the food groups. High-protein foods are emphasized more than carbohydrate foods in the Link-and-Balance Food Pyramid.

Of course, carbohydrates are not to be totally eliminated. Most carbohydrates are packed with necessary and important vitamins, minerals, and other nutrients. It is very important that you do not eliminate high-carbohydrate foods from your daily intake or restrict them too severely. Don't make up unnecessary restrictions that will only cause you to feel deprived. Whole grains, fruits, starchy vegetables, and even sugary foods have a place in a healthy diet.

Try to include all of the elements of a healthy diet every day. You need to drink plenty of water and eat adequate amounts of vegetables, protein, complex carbohydrates including fruits and grains, and a small amount of the "good" fats to keep your body in good working order.

*Figure 6.1  The Link-and-Balance Food Pyramid*

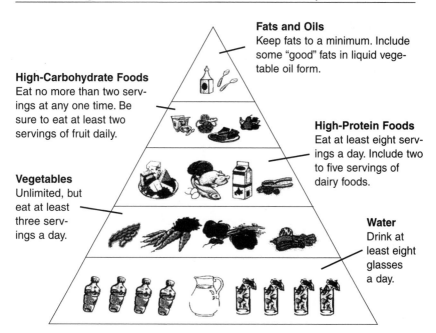

**Fats and Oils**
Keep fats to a minimum. Include some "good" fats in liquid vegetable oil form.

**High-Carbohydrate Foods**
Eat no more than two servings at any one time. Be sure to eat at least two servings of fruit daily.

**High-Protein Foods**
Eat at least eight servings a day. Include two to five servings of dairy foods.

**Vegetables**
Unlimited, but eat at least three servings a day.

**Water**
Drink at least eight glasses a day.

# 7

# Test Your Link-
# and-Balance Basics

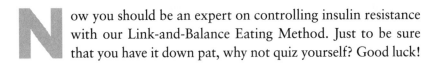ow you should be an expert on controlling insulin resistance with our Link-and-Balance Eating Method. Just to be sure that you have it down pat, why not quiz yourself? Good luck!

## *Link-and-Balance Basics*

Circle the best answer (or write it down on a separate sheet of paper if you have borrowed this book). Then, check your answers with the correct answers listed at the end of this chapter.

   1. If you have insulin resistance, the most effective way to lose weight nutritionally is to
     a. count calories
     b. count fat grams
     c. avoid eating excessive carbohydrates

   2. The best combination of foods for fat loss is
     a. low-fat, low-protein, high-carbohydrate foods
     b. low-fat foods that are not excessive in carbohydrates but have a fair amount of protein
     c. high-fat, high-protein, low-carbohydrate foods

3. Lean meats, fish, turkey, chicken, eggs, pinto beans, black beans, low-fat milk and cheese, nuts, and seeds are some of the foods that are high in
   a. protein
   b. carbohydrates
   c. salt
   d. air

4. You may eat vegetables in unlimited amounts to satisfy hunger *except* these two vegetables, which are high in starchy carbohydrates:
   a. broccoli and cauliflower
   b. lettuce and carrots
   c. corn and potatoes

5. We now know that the real culprit behind making fat if you have insulin resistance is
   a. calcium
   b. high insulin spiking
   c. eating late at night

6. High insulin spikes are caused by
   a. eating high-carbohydrate foods
   b. eating protein foods
   c. eating fatty foods

7. The big key to losing fat is to
   a. do aerobic exercises for at least ninety minutes each day
   b. eat fewer high-carbohydrate foods so that insulin is lowered
   c. eat mostly high-carbohydrate, low-calorie foods

8. How long does it take your body to actually make fat after eating excess carbohydrates?
   a. twenty-four hours
   b. only two hours
   c. a whole week

9. Carbohydrates are needed by your body for
   a. energy and brain function
   b. muscle building
   c. digestion

10. The technique of always eating protein whenever you eat carbohydrates is called
    a. fat linking
    b. food sharing
    c. protein linking

11. If you eat 30 grams of carbohydrates, you should link with how much protein?
    a. 4 grams of protein
    b. at least 14 grams of protein
    c. 7 grams of protein

12. The main job of insulin is to regulate blood glucose levels, but its other job is to
    a. store fat
    b. raise cholesterol and triglyceride levels in the blood
    c. raise blood pressure
    d. all of the above

13. If you lower your insulin spike you can
    a. lose unwanted fat
    b. normalize your blood pressure if it is too high
    c. bring down your cholesterol or triglycerides if they are too high
    d. all of the above

14. If you do not eat at regular intervals or forget to eat, you will
    a. lose weight very quickly because you will be able to keep your calories down
    b. slow down your metabolism and lose weight more slowly
    c. speed up your weight loss because your metabolism is faster

15. The three "tricks" to lowering your insulin spikes include (pick three)
    a. limit high-carbohydrate foods to no more than two servings in a two-hour interval
    b. eat high-fiber carbohydrate foods
    c. combine carbohydrates with a protein food
    d. count calories
    e. avoid eating for six- to eight-hour intervals

16. The protein linking technique to lower insulin works best when
    a. you eat protein right *before* you eat your carbohydrates
    b. you eat protein right *with* your carbohydrates
    c. both a and b

17. You may eat protein anytime, even without a carbohydrate food.

    true or false

18. Protein linking works by lowering the insulin spike as you eat carbohydrates.

    true or false

19. You may eat carbohydrates without protein.

    true or false

20. Corn and potatoes are too high in carbohydrates to be allowed on this eating method.

    true or false

21. Dairy, legumes, and vegetables do contain carbohydrates but do not cause insulin spikes; therefore they do not need to be counted in your carbohydrate limit of 30 grams.

    true or false

22. If you had to eat something from a vending machine, which one would be the best choice?

    a. potato chips
    b. licorice
    c. peanuts
    d. popcorn

23. You can avoid hypoglycemia (low blood sugar) symptoms such as intense sugar or carbohydrate cravings, headache, drowsiness after you eat, mental fogginess in the afternoon, or jitteriness by

    a. eating candy in the afternoon
    b. keeping your insulin levels from spiking throughout your day
    c. eating large amounts of pasta or bread

24. Exercising also helps you to lower insulin spikes.

    true or false

25. If you want to lose fat, you need to lower your insulin; if you want to lower your insulin, you need to lower your carbohydrates.

    true or false

## *Extra Credit: Home Pantry Assignment*

Go through some of the foods in your pantry or cabinets and look at their food labels.

1. First, check to see how many servings are contained in each package.

2. Then check how many total carbohydrate grams per serving are listed.

3. Then check how many protein grams per serving are listed.

Determine if the total carbohydrates stays within your carbohydrate budget of 30 grams in a two-hour interval. The protein grams should be at least 14 grams if there are 30 grams of carbohydrates.

**Answers**

1. c   2. b   3. a   4. c   5. b   6. a   7. b   8. b   9. a   10. c   11. b   12. d   13. d   14. b   15. a, b, c   16. c   17. true   18. true   19. false   20. false   21. true   22. c   23. b   24. true   25. true

23 or more correct: You're an expert! You understand the concept of linking and balancing well. Look over the questions that you missed to be sure you understand the rationale behind the correct answers.

20 to 22 correct: That's a good start. You are getting the hang of it! Look at the questions you missed to see if there is a common thread. If so, you may want to review the chapter or chapters that address those concepts.

19 or fewer correct: You're a beginner. You may want to review the book more carefully. If you have not looked at the link-and-balance seesaws in Chapter 4, you might want to do this now. The method may become clearer to you if you are a visual person.

By now you probably know how to link proteins with carbohydrates and balance the amount of protein to carbohydrates, and you know to keep saturated fat to a minimum. Plus you are aware of the nutrients and amount of water that you must include as part of your daily routine. You have the food lists and know how to read labels at the grocery store. In short, you are now becoming a link-and-balance master. Now the rest of the book will show you how to do it and how to keep on doing it for a lifetime.

# PART III

# Making the Method Work for You

# 8

---

# Link-and-Balance Menus
## and Recipes

You may need some ideas to get you started on a lifetime of linking and balancing. This chapter contains a few breakfast, lunch, and dinner menu ideas and plenty of recipes to go with them. You pick the ones that fit your lifestyle. Remember that your possibilities are endless. You can link and balance any foods. Also note that vegetables and foods made from vegetables can be added to any meal or snack without linking. Refer to the section in Chapter 4 on food label reading (page 59) to find out how to fit in all of your favorites.

## Breakfast Menus

Many people with insulin resistance decide to skip breakfast in order to save on calories, but doing this may actually promote fat storing. After not eating all night, your body is in a fasting metabolic state. In this state, your body will conserve and store more fat. By eating first thing in the morning or very soon after rising, you will break this fasting state and allow your body to start burning fat more efficiently.

If you are not used to eating breakfast, here are some ideas to rev up your morning metabolism engine. Create a perfectly linked-and-balanced breakfast by choosing one item from each column or two items from each column.

## Mix-and-Match Breakfasts

**High-Protein Foods**

2 tablespoons dry-roasted soy nuts

1 hard-cooked egg*

1 soft-cooked egg*

1 egg fried in nonstick oil

1 poached egg

1 scrambled egg or egg white

1 1-egg or egg white omelet

1 cup light yogurt*

1 ounce string cheese*

1 ounce reduced-fat cheese*

1 ounce fat-free cheese*

1 cup nonfat or 1% milk* (can be heated and used with coffee or sugar-free cocoa)

⅓ cup nonfat dried milk*

2 tablespoons peanut butter*

3 tablespoons nonfat cream cheese*

1 ounce low-fat sausage or ham

1 ounce low-fat Canadian bacon

**High-Carbohydrate Foods**

½ English muffin*

1 slice bread or toast*

2 slices light bread or toast*

1 slice French toast

1 4-inch waffle

1 4-inch pancake

½ cup fruit other than berries or melon (no sugar added)*

1 cup berries*

1 cup melon*

½ grapefruit*

½ banana*

½ cup no-sugar-added fruit juice*

Cold cereal (in amount to provide 15 grams of carbohydrates)*

½ cup cooked cereal

⅓ bagel*

1 minibagel*

1 small tortilla*

½ cup hashed brown potatoes

*Quick and easy to prepare

### Favorite Breakfast Combos

Egg on an English muffin with a slice of reduced-fat
    or nonfat cheese
Waffle with cottage cheese and fruit
Fruit and cottage cheese
Yogurt with Grapenuts or low-fat granola
Cold cereal with milk
Hot cereal cooked in milk or with nonfat dried milk added
⅓ bagel with nonfat cream cheese
Latte with melba toast
Toast with peanut butter
Breakfast burrito

# Lunch and Dinner Menus

The menu items below in **bold** print are one serving of recipes given later in this chapter. Add nonfat milk and/or sugar-free sodas, seltzers, or water to any of these menus. You may drink one four- to six-ounce glass of dry wine with your meal. The amount of carbohydrates in dry wines is very low and does not need to be considered in linking and balancing if you drink only one glass. However, if your goal is to lose weight, we recommend you drink no more than two glasses of wine or mixed drinks each week.

## *Meal 1*

**Pasta Primavera with Italian Sausage**
Green salad with reduced-fat or fat-free dressing
**Low-Fat Garlic-Herb Bread**
½ cup no-sugar-added ice cream or frozen yogurt

## *Meal 2*

**Chicken Enchiladas**
Nonfat, low-fat, or vegetarian refried beans
Sautéed onions and peppers

## Meal 3

**Turkey Breast Tenders Parmesan**
½ cup cooked pasta
Steamed or sautéed vegetables, such as green beans or
    zucchini
½ cup fresh fruit or canned fruit packed in juice

## Meal 4

2 ounces or more roasted turkey or chicken without skin
**Fat-Free Mashed Potatoes**
**Low-Sugar Cranberry Gelatin Salad**
**Vegetables in Buttery Herb Sauce**
1 dinner roll with reduced-fat or fat-free margarine

## Meal 5

**Chicken Breasts Dijon**
**Garlic Mashed Potatoes**
Sliced tomatoes, cucumbers, and onions in vinaigrette
    dressing
Sugar-free gelatin

## Meal 6

**Salmon with Sour Cream–Dill Sauce in Phyllo Pastry**
Mixed greens and tomato wedges with low-fat or nonfat
    dressing
**No-Sugar-Added Lime Pie**

## Meal 7

Very Low-Fat Fettuccine Alfredo
2 ounces or more cooked shrimp, scallops, or clams
Steamed broccoli
Mixed greens with nonfat or low-fat dressing
1 no-sugar-added ice cream bar

## Meal 8

Marinated London Broil with Mushroom-Wine Gravy
Vegetable kabobs (skewered onions, zucchini, peppers, and
    cherry tomatoes basted with olive oil and broiled or
    grilled)
Fat-Free Sour Cream–Chocolate Cake

## Meal 9

2 ounces low-fat deli meat, tuna, or low-fat cheese on 2 slices
    bread
Green salad with low-fat or fat-free dressing *or* other vegetable
    salad, such as Fat-Free, No-Added-Sugar Three-Bean Salad
    *or* Asian Vegetable Slaw
*or* a vegetable soup such as Black Bean Gazpacho *or* Easy Mine-
    strone Soup

## Meal 10

Fifteen-Minute Vegetarian Chili
1 two-inch-square piece corn bread with fat-free margarine or
    1 teaspoon reduced-fat margarine
Green salad with low-fat or fat-free dressing

# Appetizers

## *Low-Fat Chinese Stuffed Mushrooms*

Everyone loves stuffed mushrooms at a party! Make these high-protein appetizers ahead and refrigerate them for up to one day before baking. Then pop them in the oven so you have time to get ready before your company arrives.

>   2 cups chicken broth
>   ½ cup white cooking wine
>   40 large fresh mushrooms, stems removed
>   1 5-ounce can water chestnuts
>   1 pound low-fat breakfast sausage
>   2 tablespoons minced fresh parsley
>   2 green onions, chopped fine
>   1 tablespoon soy sauce
>   2 teaspoons ground ginger
>   ⅛ teaspoon black pepper

Heat oven to 350°F. In a deep skillet, heat broth, wine, and mushroom caps to boiling. Cover and simmer for 3 minutes. Remove from heat. Remove mushroom caps with a slotted spoon and set aside till cool; reserve liquid. Chop mushroom stems, water chestnuts, and breakfast sausage fine into a bowl. Add parsley, onions, soy sauce, ginger, and black pepper. Mix well. Stuff each mushroom cap with mixture. Arrange caps stuffed side up in a shallow baking pan. Add reserved liquid. Bake 25 minutes (or 30 minutes if mushroom caps have been chilled). Serve hot.

**Serves 20**

Nutrition information per serving:
Protein: 6 grams
Carbohydrates: 3 grams
Fat: 2 grams
Calories: 81

# Marinated Mushrooms and Artichoke Hearts

These tangy appetizers have very little carbohydrates, fat, or calories—but so much flavor!

> 1 cup white vinegar
> ½ cup red wine vinegar
> 1 teaspoon dill weed
> ¼ cup minced onion
> 2 cloves garlic, minced
> 1 teaspoon salt
> ¼ teaspoon black pepper
> 2 packets artificial sweetener (1 gram each)
> 1 pound fresh mushrooms
> 1 14-ounce can artichoke hearts in water
> 1 tablespoon chopped pimiento

Put white vinegar, red wine vinegar, dill weed, onion, garlic, salt, and black pepper into a saucepan. Bring to a boil, then cool. Stir artificial sweetener into cooled dressing. If mushrooms are large, slice or quarter them. Mix mushrooms, artichoke hearts, and pimiento into dressing in a bowl. Marinate for several hours or overnight.

**Serves 6**

Nutrition information per serving:
Protein: 3 grams
Carbohydrates: 7 grams
Fat: less than 0.5 gram
Calories: 39

# *Low-Fat Layered Bean Dip*

Take this dip to a party and you'll get requests for the recipe every time. Serve it with low-fat tortilla chips.

> 2 pounds ground beef or turkey with less than 10 percent fat or soy ground beef substitute
> 1 16-ounce can fat-free refried beans
> 1 1.5-ounce package taco seasoning
> 16 ounces fat-free sour cream
> 5 green onions, sliced
> 1 4-ounce can diced green chilies
> 3 tomatoes, diced
> 2 cups grated low-fat cheddar cheese

Brown ground beef, turkey, or soy in a frying pan. Mix in refried beans and taco seasoning. Spread meat mixture evenly in the bottom of a 13″ × 9″ baking dish. Spread sour cream on top of the meat mixture. Sprinkle over sour cream, green onions, chilies, and tomato. Top layers with cheese and serve.

**Serves 20**

Nutrition information per ½ cup serving (not including
   tortilla chips):
Protein: 14 grams
Carbohydrate: 8 grams
Fat: 7.5 grams
Calories: 163

# Soups

## *Easy Minestrone Soup*

This one-pot meal takes just minutes to put together. Serve this high-protein soup alone or linked with high-carbohydrate fruits and breads.

    1 pound extra-lean ground beef
    4 cups chicken broth
    8 ounces kidney beans
    2 cups canned tomatoes
    1 clove garlic, minced
    ¼ teaspoon black pepper
    ½ teaspoon salt
    ¼ cup dry white wine

Brown ground beef in a large stockpot or deep skillet. Add chicken broth, kidney beans, tomatoes, garlic, black pepper, salt, and white wine. Simmer 1 hour to blend flavors.

**Serves 8**

Nutrition information per 1-cup serving:
Protein: 17 grams
Carbohydrates: 10 grams
Fat: 8 grams
Calories: 205

# *Black Bean Gazpacho*

This cold summer soup is a snap to make in your food processor. There is no cooking needed; keep your kitchen cool!

2 tomatoes
¼ cucumber
¼ green pepper
2 stalks celery
¼ onion
2 16-ounce cans black beans
2 12-ounce cans vegetable juice
2 tablespoons red wine vinegar
1 teaspoon minced garlic
½ teaspoon crushed red pepper
Fat-free sour cream
Baked tortilla chips, crushed
Cilantro sprig

Dice tomatoes, cucumber, green pepper, celery, and onion in a food processor. Combine vegetables and black beans, vegetable juice, wine vinegar, garlic, and crushed red pepper. Refrigerate overnight to blend flavors. Garnish with a dollop of sour cream, crushed chips, and a cilantro sprig.

**Serves 8**

Nutrition information per serving (not including garnish):
Protein: 8 grams
Carbohydrates: 22 grams
Fat: 0 grams
Calories: 122

# *Fifteen-Minute Vegetarian Chili*

Make this chili after work—it's ready in fifteen minutes. Add cooked lean ground beef or turkey or vegetarian "beef" crumbles if you desire. Your family will love it with or without. Serve this chili with a green salad.

> 1 16-ounce can red kidney beans
> 1 16-ounce can stewed tomatoes
> ½ teaspoon garlic powder
> 1 tablespoon dehydrated onion flakes
> ⅛ teaspoon dried oregano
> ⅛ teaspoon dried basil
> 2 teaspoons chili powder
> Dash Tabasco sauce
> 1 teaspoon beef bouillon

Mix kidney beans, tomatoes, garlic powder, onion flakes, oregano, basil, chili powder, Tabasco, and bouillon in a large pot. Simmer uncovered over medium heat for 15 minutes, stirring frequently.

**Serves 4**

Nutrition information per serving:
Protein: 7 grams
Carbohydrate: 23 grams
Fat: 0 grams
Calories: 105

## Side Dishes

Most of the recipes in this section must be linked to high-protein foods.

## *Low-Fat Garlic-Herb Bread*

Use fat-free spray margarine and light French bread to make this very low-fat, low-carbohydrate garlic bread.

> 2 slices light French bread
> Fat-free liquid spray margarine
> Minced garlic
> Italian seasoning, basil, or oregano, as desired

Spray both sides of each slice of bread with spray margarine. Heat a nonstick pan. Add slices and brown each on one side. Turn slices over to brown second sides. Meanwhile, spread grilled sides with garlic and sprinkle them with herbs.

**Serves 1**

Nutrition information per serving:
Protein: 4 grams
Carbohydrates: 15 grams
Fat: 2 grams
Calories: 80

# Spinach Salad with Summer Berries and Almonds

This light and delicious salad is packed with vitamins A and C. Serve it with your favorite low-fat or fat-free dressing or **Dijon–Poppy Seed Dressing**.

12 ounces raw spinach, torn into bite-sized pieces
1 cup fresh sliced strawberries, raspberries, or diced papaya
1 ounce slivered almonds

Toss together spinach, strawberries, and almonds. Chill and serve.

**Serves 6**

Nutrition information per serving:
Protein: 2 grams
Carbohydrates: 5.5 grams
Fat: 3 grams
Calories: 46

# Dijon–Poppy Seed Dressing

Try this dressing with **Spinach Salad with Summer Berries and Almonds.**

> ⅓ cup red wine vinegar or garlic-flavored red wine vinegar
> ⅓ cup water
> 1 tablespoon Dijon mustard
> 1 teaspoon poppy seeds
> 2 packets artificial sweetener (1 gram each)
> 1 tablespoon olive oil

Mix together wine vinegar, water, mustard, poppy seeds, sweetener, and olive oil. Chill and use to dress a salad.

**Serves 9**

Nutrition information per serving:
Protein: less than 0.5 gram
Carbohydrates: less than 0.5 gram
Fat: 2 grams
Calories: 16

# Low-Sugar Cranberry Gelatin Salad

This recipe makes a beautiful gelatin salad to serve during holiday festivities. Or serve it with poultry instead of high-carbohydrate cranberry sauce.

> 2 cups raw cranberries
> 1 orange
> 1 6-ounce can crushed pineapple in juice
> Hot water
> 2 0.3-ounce packages sugar-free raspberry gelatin
> ½ cup diced celery

Wash cranberries and the orange. In a food processor, finely grind cranberries and the whole orange including the rind. Add pineapple with juice. Separate juices from fruit and set fruit mixture aside. Mix juices with enough hot water to make 2 cups. Dissolve gelatin in juice mixture. Chill in refrigerator till slightly gelled. Stir fruit mixture and celery into gelatin mixture and pour all into a mold. Refrigerate till well set. Unmold and serve.

**Serves 6**

Nutrition information per serving:
Protein: less than 1 gram
Carbohydrates: 13 grams
Fat: 0 grams
Calories: 65

# Asian Vegetable Slaw

Seasoned rice wine vinegar, soy sauce, sesame oil, and bean sprouts give this coleslaw an Asian flair.

> 1 head green cabbage, shredded
> 6 carrots, shredded
> ⅓ pound bean sprouts
> ¼ cup rice wine vinegar
> 2 tablespoons soy sauce
> 1 tablespoon canola or olive oil
> 1 teaspoon sesame oil
> 2 packets artificial sweetener (1 gram each)
> ¼ cup water
> ¼ teaspoon black pepper

Place cabbage and carrots in a large bowl. Rinse and drain bean sprouts and stir into cabbage mixture. Combine vinegar, soy sauce, canola oil, sesame oil, sweetener, water, and black pepper in a jar with a tightly fitting lid; shake to blend. Pour dressing over cabbage mixture and toss gently to combine. Cover and chill.

**Serves 10**

Nutrition information per serving:
Protein: 2 grams
Carbohydrates: 10 grams
Fat: 2 grams
Calories: 63

# Curried Fruit Compote

Fruit canned in juice instead of syrup has a lower carbohydrate content. This is an exotic side dish to serve with meat. Or use it as a topping for no-sugar-added ice cream or yogurt for an interesting dessert.

> 1 16-ounce can peach halves in juice
> 1 16-ounce can pear halves in juice
> 1 16-ounce can pineapple slices in juice
> ¼ cup fat-free liquid margarine
> 2 teaspoons curry powder
> Artificial sweetener

Preheat oven to 350°F. Drain peach halves, pear halves, and pineapple slices well. Arrange fruit in a 2-quart baking dish. Mix margarine and curry powder in a small bowl; pour over fruit. Bake for 30 minutes. Sprinkle with artificial sweetener to taste. Serve hot.

**Serves 8**

Nutrition information per serving:
Protein: 0 grams
Carbohydrates: 24 grams
Fat: 0 grams
Calories: 73

# Fat-Free Potato Salad

Adding hard-cooked eggs to this picnic favorite increases the protein. You'll still need to link it with some extra protein—perhaps a barbecued lean steak or chicken breast.

12 eggs
4 large white potatoes
6 green onions
2 dill pickles
6 radishes
¾ cup fat-free mayonnaise
2 tablespoons mustard
2 teaspoons white vinegar
½ teaspoon salt

Cook eggs until hard-cooked, about 10 minutes, and potatoes until just tender, in boiling water. Chill. Peel potatoes, if desired, and cut into bite-sized pieces. Dice eggs. Finely chop the green onions, pickles, and radishes. In a small bowl blend mayonnaise, mustard, vinegar, and salt. Gently stir together potatoes, eggs, and mayonnaise mixture in a large bowl. Chill at least 2 hours before serving.

**Serves 18**

Nutrition information per serving:
Protein: 4 grams
Carbohydrates: 15 grams
Fat: less than 1 gram
Calories: 76

# Garlic Mashed Potatoes

The instant mashed potatoes make this recipe quick. But if you'd like to use fresh, cook 1½ pounds peeled potatoes in boiling water till soft and omit boiling water. Either way, be sure to link and balance these potatoes with protein.

> 4 cloves garlic, unpeeled
> 1½ cups boiling water
> ⅓ cup fat-free sour cream
> 2 tablespoons fat-free liquid margarine
> ½ teaspoon salt
> 1⅓ cups instant mashed potatoes

Microwave garlic on high 30 seconds, and then press cloves with the flat side of a knife to remove the skin. Mash garlic with a fork in a large bowl. Add boiling water, sour cream, liquid margarine, salt, and instant mashed potatoes and stir. Cover and let stand 30 seconds. Whip with a fork; serve.

**Serves 3**

Nutrition information per serving:
Protein: 4 grams
Carbohydrates: 27 grams
Fat: 0 grams
Calories: 124

# *Fat-Free Mashed Potatoes*

Potatoes are naturally low in fat and high in flavor. Why add fat and calories to them? Be sure you do serve them with a food that is high in protein, though, to link and balance with the natural carbohydrates in this vegetable.

> 2 pounds white potatoes
> ½ cup fat-free sour cream
> 2 tablespoons fat-free liquid margarine
> ½ teaspoon salt
> Dash black pepper
> Skim milk
> Paprika, snipped parsley, or chives

Wash potatoes and remove eyes. Peel if desired. Cut into large pieces. Heat salted water 1 inch deep in saucepan to boiling. Add potatoes. Cover and heat again to boiling. Cook potatoes until tender, 30 to 35 minutes. Drain. Mash potatoes until smooth. Add sour cream, margarine, salt, and black pepper and beat until potatoes are light and fluffy. (Add some skim milk if necessary.) If desired, garnish with paprika, snipped parsley, or chives.

**Serves 5**

Nutrition information per serving:
Protein: 4 grams
Carbohydrates: 28 grams
Fat: 0 grams
Calories: 127

# Fat-Free Hashed Brown Potatoes

Enjoy this low-fat version of an old favorite with eggs or breakfast meats. You may use preshredded fresh, frozen, or dehydrated hashed brown potatoes.

> Nonstick spray oil
> 3 cups shredded potatoes
> 2 tablespoons dried onion flakes
> 2 tablespoons dried parsley flakes
> 1 cup chicken broth
> Butter-flavored granules, spray, or sprinkles

Spray a nonstick pan with spray oil. Add potatoes, onion flakes, parsley flakes, and chicken broth. Cook uncovered over medium heat until most liquid has evaporated. Continue to cook until hashed brown potatoes are brown on one side. Gently turn over. Cook till browned on the other side. Season with butter flavoring to taste.

**Serves 6**

Nutrition information per serving:
Protein: 2 grams
Carbohydrates: 17 grams
Fat: 0 grams
Calories: 72

# Buttery-Flavored Dilled Potatoes and Green Beans

Use fat-free liquid margarine to give these potatoes a buttery flavor. Canned potatoes and green beans make this a quick and easy side dish.

1 16-ounce can whole baby potatoes
1 16-ounce can green beans *or* 16 ounces frozen green beans, thawed
1 tablespoon minced onion flakes
2 tablespoons very hot water
2 tablespoons fat-free liquid margarine
2 tablespoons lemon juice
1 teaspoon dill weed

Drain potatoes and green beans. Rehydrate onions in hot water for several minutes. Heat potatoes, green beans, onion flakes, liquid margarine, lemon juice, and dill weed thoroughly in a nonstick pan and serve.

**Serves 4**

Nutrition information per serving:
Protein: 2 grams
Carbohydrates: 16 grams
Fat: less than 1 gram
Calories: 69

# *Apples and Sweet Potatoes*

Sweet potatoes are a good source of vitamin A, an important nutrient. This casserole is a better substitute for higher-carbohydrate sweet potato dishes made with simple sugars.

Salt
2 pounds sweet potatoes or yams
2 tart apples
1 tablespoon cornstarch
1 teaspoon salt
¼ teaspoon pumpkin pie spice
1 cup apple juice

Heat salted water in a saucepan to boiling (use enough water to cover potatoes). Add potatoes and boil 30 minutes. Meanwhile, slice and core apples. Heat oven to 350°F. Drain, peel, and slice sweet potatoes. Arrange apples and sweet potatoes in an ungreased 1½-quart casserole. In a small saucepan, stir together cornstarch, salt, pumpkin pie spice, and apple juice. Cook, stirring constantly, until mixture thickens and boils. Boil and stir 1 minute. Pour over sweet potatoes and apples. Cover. Bake 1 hour.

**Serves 6**

Nutrition information per serving:
Protein: 2 grams
Carbohydrates: 29 grams
Fat: 0 grams
Calories: 125

# Vegetables in Buttery Herb Sauce

Using fat-free liquid margarine decreases the fat and calories of traditional buttered vegetables but gives you the same buttery flavor.

1½ pounds fresh carrots, zucchini, or green beans, sliced
¼ cup fat-free liquid margarine
¼ teaspoon seasoned salt
⅛ teaspoon black pepper
1 tablespoon chopped onion
¼ teaspoon dried dill weed, basil, or tarragon

Cook carrots, zucchini, or green beans till barely tender (don't overcook). Drain; return to pan. Add liquid margarine, seasoned salt, black pepper, onion, and dill weed, basil, or tarragon. Heat through.

**Serves 6**

Nutrition information per serving:
Protein: less than 1 gram
Carbohydrates: 4 grams
Fat: 0 grams
Calories: 15

# Fat-Free, No-Added-Sugar Three-Bean Salad

Use artificial sweetener instead of sugar and leave out the oil in this recipe for a veggie treat that is so tasty you won't believe it is so good for you. Rice wine vinegar gives it a mild flavor.

> 1 16-ounce can cut green beans (drained)
> 1 16-ounce can wax beans (drained)
> 1 16-ounce can kidney beans (drained)
> 1 cup seasoned rice wine vinegar
> 1½ ounces chopped pimiento
> 2 packets artificial sweetener (1 gram each)
> ¼ teaspoon Mrs. Dash seasoning
> 1 teaspoon minced garlic
> ⅛ teaspoon dried dill weed or tarragon (optional)
> 1 tablespoon chopped fresh onion

Stir together green beans, wax beans, kidney beans, vinegar, pimiento, sweetener, Mrs. Dash, garlic, dill, and onion. Chill several hours. Serve.

**Serves 10**

Nutrition information per serving:
Protein: 5 grams
Carbohydrates: 15 grams
Fat: less than 1 gram
Calories: 82

# Mushroom Pilaf

Rice is a high-carbohydrate food but can be part of a healthy diet if you serve it as a side dish for a high-protein main course. It's naturally low in fat as long as you don't add fat in the form of margarine or oil. Brown rice is higher in nutrients and fiber but will take longer to cook—increase simmering time to fifty minutes.

> 1 4-ounce can sliced mushrooms (undrained)
> 1 teaspoon dried parsley flakes
> ½ teaspoon seasoned salt
> 2 teaspoons minced onion
> ⅛ teaspoon black pepper
> 1 cup rice
> 2 cups beef or chicken broth

Place mushrooms, parsley, seasoned salt, onion, black pepper, rice, and broth in a saucepan. Heat to boiling. Reduce heat; simmer 25 to 30 minutes. Fluff pilaf with a fork before serving.

**Serves 9**

Nutrition information per serving:
Protein: 2.5 grams
Carbohydrates: 31 grams
Fat: less than 0.5 gram
Calories: 136

# Kashi-Lentil Pilaf

You can find kashi in the cereal or health food section of most grocery stores. It is a very high-protein grain product. Combined with lentils, which are also high in protein, it makes a terrific pilaf for those with insulin resistance. Use multicolored lentils for an attractive color.

> ½ cup dried lentils
> 3 cups water
> 3 teaspoons chicken broth
> 1 cup kashi
> 2 ounces canned sliced mushrooms
> 2 teaspoons canned diced green chilies
> ½ teaspoon garlic powder
> 1 teaspoon salt-free all-purpose seasoning

Rinse lentils. In a large pot, combine lentils, water, and chicken broth. Bring to a boil over high heat. Add kashi. Cook covered over medium heat (not simmering), 25 minutes. Add mushrooms, chilies, garlic powder, and all-purpose seasoning and serve.

**Serves 6**

Nutrition information per serving:
Protein: 7 grams
Carbohydrates: 27 grams
Fat: 2.5 grams
Calories: 145

# Easy, Cheesy, Low-Fat Noodles Romanoff

Here's a way to add protein to and reduce fat in a traditionally high-fat, high-carbohydrate side dish. And it's all done on the stovetop.

> 6 ounces noodles (uncooked)
> ¼ cup minced fresh onion
> ½ cup fat-free cottage cheese
> ½ cup fat-free sour cream
> ⅛ teaspoon garlic powder
> ¼ teaspoon seasoned salt
> ½ teaspoon Worcestershire sauce
> Dash Tabasco sauce
> ⅛ cup grated fat-free Parmesan cheese
> Parsley flakes

Cook noodles according to package directions. Drain, rinse, and return noodles to pot. Add onion, cottage cheese, sour cream, garlic powder, seasoned salt, Worcestershire sauce, Tabasco, and Parmesan cheese. Heat on low till heated through (being careful not to let noodle mixture burn). Garnish with parsley flakes if desired.

**Serves 5**

Nutrition information per serving:
Protein: 8 grams
Carbohydrate: 28 grams
Fat: 0.5 gram
Calories: 158

# *Very Low-Fat Fettuccine Alfredo*

Fettuccine alfredo that is almost fat free? What a dream come true! Try adding fried pieces of thinly sliced 99 percent fat-free ham for a carbonara or clams for a clam sauce. Be sure to serve this dish with a high-protein food to link and balance it, perhaps sautéed shrimp or chicken.

> 5 ounces fettuccine (uncooked)
> 2 teaspoons minced garlic
> ¼ cup minced fresh onion
> ¼ cup dry white wine
> 1½ tablespoons flour
> 1 cup evaporated skim milk
> ½ teaspoon dried basil
> 1 teaspoon dried parsley flakes
> Butter-flavored granules or powder
> Salt
> Black pepper
> ¾ cup grated fat-free Parmesan cheese

Cook fettuccine according to package directions. Drain, rinse, and set aside. Sauté garlic and onion in wine until onion is clear. In a separate bowl or cup, stir together flour and evaporated milk until smooth. Add milk mixture to onion mixture. Cook over medium heat, stirring frequently, until thick and bubbly. Add basil, parsley, and butter flavor, salt, and black pepper to taste. Toss with fettuccine. Sprinkle with Parmesan cheese.

**Serves 5**

Nutrition information per serving:
Protein: 8 grams
Carbohydrates: 31 grams
Fat: 1 gram
Calories: 174

# Main Dishes

The recipes in this section are high in protein with very little carbohydrates other than those that are in vegetables, dairy, or legumes. Link them with any high-carbohydrate food.

## *Salmon Poached in Wine*

This recipe is so easy and so delicious. It also works with other fish.

> 1 cup white wine
> ½ cup water
> 1 bay leaf
> ½ teaspoon peppercorns
> 4 ½-inch-thick salmon steaks or fillets
> 4 slices onion
> 8 slices lemon

Bring wine, water, bay leaf, and peppercorns to a boil in a covered skillet. Add salmon. Top each fillet with one slice onion and one slice lemon. Cover; simmer 8 minutes or until salmon flakes easily with a fork. Remove salmon with a slotted spoon to a serving plate. Garnish with 4 lemon slices.

**Serves 4**

Nutrition information per serving:
Protein: 28 grams
Carbohydrates: 3 grams
Fat: 7 grams
Calories: 187

# Grilled Shrimp in Spicy Thai Marinade

Grill a skewer of vegetables such as red and green peppers and onions along with the shrimp. The finished grilled shrimp and vegetables make a wonderful salad topping for an easy summer meal. This marinade can be used for grilled poultry or pork as well. If you're using bamboo skewers, soak them at least one hour to keep them from burning.

> 1 jalapeño or other hot pepper
> ¼ cup soy sauce
> 2 tablespoons lime juice
> 1 tablespoon minced garlic
> ½ teaspoon ground ginger
> ½ teaspoon sesame oil
> 1 pound jumbo shrimp (8 to 15 per pound), peeled
>     and deveined

Remove seeds from hot pepper. Slice into strips. Place hot pepper, soy sauce, lime juice, garlic, ginger, sesame oil, and shrimp in a large resealable plastic bag or covered bowl. Marinate sealed bag or covered bowl in the refrigerator for 30 minutes to 24 hours. Thread marinated shrimp onto barbecue skewers. Grill shrimp 5 to 8 minutes, turning frequently, till opaque but still moist.

**Serves 4**

Nutrition information per serving:
Protein: 23 grams
Carbohydrates: 1 gram
Fat: 2.5 grams
Calories: 125

# Chicken Breasts Dijon

Break away from the everyday dinner with a new way to cook skinless, boneless chicken breasts. Breading and then broiling them keeps them low in fat. The breading counts as one serving of a high-carbohydrate food.

> 2 tablespoons Dijon mustard
> 2 tablespoons minced garlic
> 1 teaspoon dried tarragon
> 1/8 teaspoon seasoned salt
> 4 skinless, boneless chicken breasts
> 3/4 cup bread crumbs
> Nonstick spray oil

Heat broiler. Mix mustard, garlic, tarragon, and seasoned salt in a wide, shallow dish. Roll chicken breasts in spice mixture, then in bread crumbs. Coat a baking dish or pan with spray oil; arrange chicken breasts in the baking dish. Broil chicken 4 inches from heat for 5 minutes. Lower heat in oven to 400°F. Place baking dish on the lower oven rack and bake 10 minutes.

**Serves 4**

Nutrition information per serving:
Protein: 24 grams
Carbohydrates: 14 grams
Fat: 5 grams
Calories: 263

# Sweet and Spicy Italian-Style Turkey Sausage

Throw in an apple to make this sausage sweet, crushed red pepper to make it spicy, and fennel seed to make it distinctively Italian! These sausages can also be made into links or crumbled and browned and used in Italian recipes.

1 small apple
1⅓ pounds ground turkey breast
2 tablespoons dried onion flakes
¼ cup egg substitute *or* 1 egg white
1 tablespoon dried parsley flakes
1 teaspoon black pepper
Dash Tabasco sauce
½ teaspoon onion powder
½ teaspoon dried oregano
1 teaspoon fennel seed
1 teaspoon crushed red pepper
Nonstick spray oil

Peel and core apple and chop fine. Mix apple, ground turkey, onion flakes, egg substitute, parsley, black pepper, Tabasco, onion powder, oregano, fennel, and red pepper together in a bowl and refrigerate at least 1 hour. Form sausage into patties. Coat a nonstick pan with spray oil. Brown patties on both sides. Cover and cook till no longer pink in the center.

**Serves 10**

Nutrition information per serving:
Protein: 14 grams
Carbohydrates: 2 grams
Fat: 0 grams
Calories: 66

# Smoky Turkey Sausage Patties

Ground turkey breast makes these breakfast sausages low in fat. Maple and smoke flavorings and apples make them moist and delicious.

> 1 pound 97 percent lean turkey ham
> 1 small apple
> 1⅓ pounds ground turkey breast
> 2 teaspoons poultry seasoning
> ½ teaspoon Mapleine
> 1 teaspoon Liquid Smoke flavor
> 1 teaspoon Kitchen Bouquet (optional)
> Nonstick spray oil

Grind turkey ham fine in a food processor and place in a large bowl. Peel and core apple. Grind apple coarse in the food processor. Add apple and ground turkey, poultry seasoning, Mapleine, Liquid Smoke, and Kitchen Bouquet, if desired, to ham; mix well. Refrigerate 1 hour; form into patties. Coat a nonstick pan with spray oil. Brown patties on both sides. Cover and cook until no longer pink in the center.

**Serves 14**

Nutrition information per serving:
Protein: 14 grams
Carbohydrates: 2 grams
Fat: 2 grams
Calories: 82

# Marinated London Broil

Slice the London broil very thin. Serve this recipe with **Mushroom-Wine Gravy.**

> ½ cup red cooking wine
> 2 tablespoons red wine vinegar
> 4 teaspoons soy sauce
> 1 teaspoon salt
> 1 teaspoon black pepper
> 4 cloves garlic, minced
> 48 ounces London broil or sirloin steak

Put cooking wine, wine vinegar, soy sauce, salt, black pepper, and garlic in a resealable plastic bag or a covered bowl and mix well. Marinate meat in the refrigerator 6 hours. Heat broiler. Broil meat 6 inches from heating element, turning and basting once with marinade, for 20 minutes for medium rare. Slice very thin and serve.

**Serves 12**

Nutrition information per serving:
Protein: 28 grams
Carbohydrates: 0 grams
Fat: 8 grams
Calories: 217

# Mushroom-Wine Gravy

Serve this gravy with **Marinated London Broil** or any other meat.

> 1 cup beef broth
> 2 teaspoons dried onion flakes
> 1 3-ounce can mushrooms
> 1½ tablespoons cornstarch
> ⅓ cup red cooking wine
> Salt
> Black pepper

In a saucepan, heat broth, onion flakes, and mushrooms to boiling; lower heat. In a separate bowl, stir cornstarch into wine till smooth. Add to beef broth mixture. Bring gravy to boil over medium heat. Boil, stirring, 2 minutes. Season with salt and black pepper to taste.

**Serves 6**

Nutrition information per serving:
Protein: less than 1 gram
Carbohydrates: 7 grams
Fat: less than 1 gram
Calories: 25

# Pasta Salad

Make this summertime favorite in no time. Fat-free cheese adds protein.

> 6 ounces pasta
> ½ red onion
> 2 green peppers
> 2 tomatoes
> 6 ounces fat-free mozzarella cheese
> 2 heads broccoli
> 1½ ounces dry sun-dried tomatoes
> Hot water
> 6 (fluid) ounces fat-free Italian dressing

Cook pasta according to package directions; drain, rinse, and chill. Slice onion thin. Dice green peppers, tomatoes, and cheese. Cut broccoli into florets and then into small pieces. Rehydrate sun-dried tomatoes by soaking them in hot water for 1 minute. Toss together pasta, onion, green pepper, tomato, mozzarella, broccoli, sun-dried tomatoes, and Italian dressing. Chill 2 hours before serving.

**Serves 12**

Nutrition information per serving:
Protein: 8 grams
Carbohydrates: 18 grams
Fat: 1 gram
Calories: 107

# *Basic Quiche with Potato Crust*

Using already-shredded hashed brown potatoes will speed up your cooking time. For variety, you may add any of the following fillings: finely diced 97 percent fat-free ham, imitation bacon bits, canned or cooked crab or shrimp, sautéed vegetables such as onions, broccoli, red or green peppers, and mushrooms.

> Nonstick spray oil
> ½ pound shredded potatoes
> ¼ teaspoon salt
> 6 egg whites *or* 1½ cups egg substitute
> 1 cup skim milk
> 1 tablespoon sherry
> ⅛ teaspoon white pepper
> ⅛ teaspoon nutmeg
> 4 ounces shredded low-fat cheddar cheese
> 1 ounce grated fat-free Parmesan cheese

Arrange oven rack in center position. Heat oven to 400°F. Coat a pie pan with nonstick spray. Press the shredded potatoes into the pie pan. Bake 12 minutes. Remove potato crust from the oven and set aside.

Lower oven temperature to 375°F. Mix together salt, egg whites, milk, sherry, white pepper, and nutmeg; set aside. Place cheddar cheese (and any optional fillings) into the partially baked potato crust. Pour egg mixture over cheese (it's OK if it goes over the top of the potatoes). Sprinkle Parmesan cheese over the top. Bake 35 minutes. Serve hot or cold.

**Serves 6**

Nutrition information per serving:
Protein: 14.5 grams
Carbohydrates: 14 grams
Fat: 1 gram
Calories: 131

# Stir-Fry Vegetables and Tofu in Peanut Sauce

Peanut butter gives this tofu a meaty flavor. Serve this dish with rice or noodles if you desire.

> 1 10½-ounce package firm tofu
> ¼ cup soy sauce
> Nonstick spray oil
> 1 large onion, cut into wedges
> 1 pound fresh or frozen stir-fry vegetables (such as celery, carrots, broccoli, red or green peppers, and pea pods)
> ½ cup chicken broth
> 1 tablespoon peanut butter
> ¼ cup vinegar
> 3 tablespoons soy sauce
> ¼ teaspoon cayenne pepper
> ¼ teaspoon ground ginger
> 4 cloves garlic, minced
> 2 teaspoons cornstarch

Drain and rinse tofu. Slice into ½-inch cubes. Marinate in soy sauce. Meanwhile, coat a nonstick pan or wok with spray oil. Brown onion in pan. Add stir-fry vegetables. Cover and steam until almost tender. Set aside in a serving bowl.

Wipe pan or wok. Spray again with spray oil. Drain tofu. Heat pan, add tofu, and cook, turning pieces gently, until browned. Add vegetables. In a separate bowl, combine chicken broth, peanut butter, vinegar, soy sauce, cayenne, ginger, garlic, and cornstarch. Add to tofu and vegetables. Cook, stirring often, until sauce is clear and bubbly.

**Serves 6**

Nutrition information per serving:
Protein: 14 grams
Carbohydrates: 10.5 grams
Fat: 8.3 grams
Calories: 173

# Spinach and Tofu Lasagna

This lasagna uses tofu to cut down on the cheese in this tasty version of an old favorite.

> 4 ounces lasagna noodles
> 1 bunch fresh spinach *or* 1 10-ounce package frozen spinach
> Nonstick spray oil
> ¼ cup minced fresh onion
> 1 clove garlic, minced
> 1 tablespoon chopped fresh parsley
> 1 pound tofu
> 16 ounces tomato sauce
> 6 ounces shredded low-fat mozzarella cheese

Heat oven to 350°F. Cook the lasagna noodles according to package directions. If using fresh spinach, cut it into small pieces and cook it briefly in a small amount of water. If using frozen spinach, thaw and drain it well. Coat a nonstick pan with nonstick spray. Sauté the onion in the pan. Combine the spinach, onion, garlic, parsley, and tofu; mash well. Spread a ½-cup layer of tomato sauce in the bottom of a lasagna pan. Top sauce with ⅓ of the lasagna noodles. Top noodles with ½ of the tofu mixture and then with 2 ounces cheese. Repeat layering starting again with tomato sauce. Finish with a third layer of noodles followed by tomato sauce and cheese. Cover and bake 30 minutes. Uncover and bake 10 more minutes.

**Serves 4**

Nutrition information per serving:
Protein: 20 grams
Carbohydrates: 28 grams
Fat: 4 grams
Calories: 224

# Spiced Couscous with Curry Tofu

Many stores offer flavored tofu. If yours does not, use regular firm tofu. Tofu adds protein to this Middle Eastern–flavored dish, which is so easy that anyone who can boil water can make it.

2½ cups chicken broth
½ teaspoon curry powder
½ teaspoon ground cinnamon
½ cup raisins
1 tablespoon dried onion flakes
½ teaspoon minced garlic
1⅓ cups couscous
1 pound curry-flavored tofu, diced

Heat chicken broth, curry, cinnamon, raisins, onion flakes, and garlic to boiling over high heat. Add couscous and tofu; stir. Cover and let stand, unheated, 5 minutes before serving.

**Serves 4**

Nutrition information per serving:
Protein: 14 grams
Carbohydrates: 15 grams
Fat: 8 grams
Calories: 190

# Salmon with Sour Cream–Dill Sauce in Phyllo Pastry

Your guests will never know that this elegant main course is low in fat and calories.

> Nonstick spray oil or butter-flavored spray
> ½ cup fat-free sour cream
> ½ teaspoon dried dill weed
> ½ teaspoon lemon juice
> Dash Worcestershire sauce
> ⅛ teaspoon seasoned salt
> Dash Tabasco sauce
> 2 4-ounce salmon fillets
> Capers
> Chopped green onions
> 2 sheets phyllo pastry

Heat oven to 350°F. Coat a baking sheet with spray oil or butter-flavored spray. Mix sour cream, dill, lemon juice, Worcestershire sauce, seasoned salt, and Tabasco. Spread 2 tablespoons of sauce over each salmon fillet. Top with capers and green onions, if desired. Fold each sheet of phyllo in half. Spray with spray oil. Place 1 salmon fillet in the center of 1 phyllo sheet, toppings down. Fold the phyllo around the salmon like an envelope. Repeat. Place phyllo envelopes with the folded edges down on the baking sheet. Spray tops with spray oil or butter-flavored spray. Bake 40 minutes. Serve with remaining sauce.

**Serves 2**

Nutrition information per serving:
Protein: 25 grams
Carbohydrates: 15 grams
Fat: 7 grams
Calories: 279

# Turkey Breast Tenders Parmesan

Turkey tenders are quick to prepare and very low in fat. This dish goes well with pasta or steamed vegetables.

> 1 pound turkey breast
> Nonstick spray oil
> Seasoned salt
> 1 cup low-fat spaghetti sauce
> ¼ cup shredded fat-free mozzarella cheese
> ¼ cup grated fat-free Parmesan cheese

Slice turkey breast into ½-inch-thick tenders. Coat a nonstick skillet with spray oil. Brown turkey slices on both sides. Add seasoned salt to taste. Spoon spaghetti sauce onto each slice. Sprinkle with mozzarella cheese and Parmesan cheese. Cover; cook on low heat till turkey is no longer pink (do not overcook).

**Serves 4**

Nutrition information per serving:
Protein: 29 grams
Carbohydrates: 0 grams
Fat: 3 grams
Calories: 184

# Pasta Primavera with Italian Sausage

This pasta variation uses Italian turkey sausage as a low-fat protein source as well as fresh vegetables and spices. Enjoy it with wine if you like.

6 ounces spaghetti or other pasta
Nonstick spray oil
6 Italian turkey sausage links
16 ounces frozen broccoli, carrot, and cauliflower vegetable blend
½ cup sliced fresh zucchini
½ cup sliced fresh yellow squash
1 16-ounce can diced tomatoes, drained
2 tablespoons dry white cooking wine
2 tablespoons minced fresh parsley
1½ teaspoons chopped fresh basil
5 ounces grated fat-free Parmesan cheese

Cook pasta according to package directions; drain and set aside. Coat a nonstick skillet with spray oil. Brown sausages in skillet over medium heat. Add frozen vegetables, zucchini, yellow squash, canned tomatoes, and wine. Cover and cook 15 to 20 minutes or until sausages are no longer pink in the center and vegetables are tender. Toss pasta with sausage mixture and parsley, basil, and Parmesan. Serve immediately.

**Serves 6**

Nutrition information per serving:
Protein: 13 grams
Carbohydrates: 21 grams
Fat: 3.4 grams
Calories: 203

# Stir-Fry Vegetables with Chicken

Dinner will be on the table in less than fifteen minutes with this convenient entree. Serve with a half cup of instant rice for a perfect balance.

> Nonstick spray oil
> 1 pound chicken breast strips
> 1 16-ounce package frozen stir-fry vegetables
> ½ cup bottled stir-fry sauce

Coat a nonstick pan with spray oil. Add chicken. Cook about 5 minutes, until chicken is no longer pink in the middle, stirring often. Add vegetables. Cook till vegetables are tender. Add stir-fry sauce. Heat through and serve.

**Serves 6**

Nutrition information per serving:
Protein: 20.5 grams
Carbohydrates: 12 grams
Fat: 1 gram
Calories: 144

# Chicken Enchiladas

Try this quick, low-fat version of a family favorite.

> 2 10.75-ounce cans reduced-fat cream of mushroom soup
> 1 4-ounce can diced green chilies
> 2 teaspoons dried onion flakes
> 2 6-ounce cans white chicken meat
> 10 white-corn tortillas
> 1⅛ cups fat-free sour cream

Heat oven to 400°F. Mix mushroom soup, chilies, and onion flakes in a bowl. In another bowl, mix ¼ of soup mixture with chicken. Spread another ¼ of soup mixture in the bottom of a casserole dish. Place ¼ cup of the chicken mixture in the center of each tortilla. Roll up tortillas and place enchiladas edge side down in the casserole dish. Spoon remaining ½ of sauce over enchiladas. Cover and bake 10 minutes or until heated through. Serve each enchilada with 2 tablespoons sour cream.

**Serves 10**

Nutrition information per serving:
Protein: 15.5 grams
Carbohydrates: 18 grams
Fat: 5 grams
Calories: 189

# Au Gratin Potatoes with Ham

Dress up a boxed potato dish and make it a linked and balanced meal by adding ham and shredded cheese.

> 1 9-ounce box au gratin potatoes
> 2¾ cups boiling water
> 1 large onion, sliced thin
> 1 pound 99 percent fat-free ham, cut into bite-sized pieces
> 1 cup skim milk
> ½ cup shredded fat-free cheddar cheese

Heat oven to 400°F. Place potato slices and sauce mix from box and boiling water into an ungreased 2½-quart casserole dish. Add onion, ham, and milk to potato mixture and stir well. Bake uncovered 35 minutes. Sprinkle cheddar cheese over top. Bake 5 minutes more. Let stand 5 minutes before serving.

**Serves 7**

Nutrition information per serving:
Protein: 15 grams
Carbohydrates: 27.5 grams
Fat: 3.5 grams
Calories: 208

# Desserts

## *Fat-Free Pumpkin Custard*

Pumpkin provides vitamin A. Egg whites and evaporated skim milk provide protein. (But you will still need more protein to link and balance this dessert.) The combination makes this a very healthy dessert!

½ cup sugar
½ teaspoon salt
¼ teaspoon ground cloves
1 teaspoon ground cinnamon
½ teaspoon ground ginger
3 egg whites *or* ½ cup egg substitute
1 13-ounce can pumpkin
1 6-ounce can evaporated skim milk
Nonstick spray oil

Preheat oven to 425°F. Combine sugar, salt, cloves, cinnamon, ginger, and egg whites or egg substitute in a medium-sized bowl. Stir in pumpkin and evaporated milk. Mix well. Coat a casserole dish with spray oil. Pour in pumpkin mixture. Bake 15 minutes. Reduce temperature to 350°F. Bake 40 to 50 minutes. Cool.

**Serves 10**

Nutrition information per serving:
Protein: 2.5 grams
Carbohydrates: 16 grams
Fat: 0 grams
Calories: 73

# No-Sugar-Added Lime Pie

This dessert can be made with your favorite flavor of sugar-free gelatin. It is so easy to make and so delicious that your friends and family will never know it is low in carbohydrates, high in protein, and low in fat!

> 3 full sheets graham crackers
> Nonstick spray oil
> 1 3-ounce box sugar-free lime gelatin, or other flavor
> ⅔ cup boiling water
> 1 cup fat-free cottage cheese
> 8 ounces fat-free cream cheese
> 8 ounces fat-free whipped topping

In a blender or food processor, crush graham crackers into fine crumbs. Coat a pie tin with spray oil. Sprinkle crumbs into the pie tin. In the blender or processor, combine gelatin and boiling water. Process till gelatin is dissolved. Add cottage cheese and cream cheese and process until smooth. Pour pie filling into a large bowl. Fold in whipped topping. Pour into pie tin. Chill 4 hours.

**Serves 8**

Nutrition information per serving:
Protein: 9.8 grams
Carbohydrates: 17 grams
Fat: 0.5 gram
Calories: 115

# *Fat-Free Sour Cream–Chocolate Cake*

This cake uses fat-free sour cream instead of oil to keep fat and carbohydrates low but moistness high. Topped with fat-free chocolate–cream cheese frosting, this cake is sure to be a hit. Be sure to link and balance.

| Cake | Frosting |
|---|---|
| 2 cups flour | 1¼ cups cold skim milk |
| 1½ cups sugar | 4 ounces fat-free cream |
| ½ cup cocoa powder | cheese, softened |
| 2 teaspoons baking soda | 1 1-ounce box sugar-free |
| 1 cup fat-free sour cream | chocolate pudding |
| 1 cup skim milk | 8 ounces fat-free |
| 1 tablespoon vinegar | whipped topping |
| 2 teaspoons vanilla extract | |
| Nonstick spray oil | |

Preheat oven to 350°F. To make the cake batter, combine flour, sugar, cocoa, and baking soda. Add sour cream, milk, vinegar, and vanilla; mix only till blended (do not overmix). Coat a 9″ × 13″ pan with spray oil. Pour batter into pan. Bake 30 to 35 minutes or until a toothpick inserted in the center comes out clean. Cool to room temperature.

To make the frosting, blend milk and cream cheese in a food processor. Add pudding mix. Blend 2 minutes. Fold pudding mixture into whipped topping in a separate bowl. Chill. Frost cooled cake and then refrigerate until ready to serve.

**Serves 20**

Nutrition information per serving (including frosting):
Protein: 4.4 grams
Carbohydrates: 32 grams
Fat: 0 grams
Calories: 147

# Chocolate Mousse

This quick and easy dessert is high in protein and low in carbohydrates, fat, and calories. Serve it in a parfait glass.

8 ounces fat-free cottage cheese
8 ounces fat-free cream cheese
1¼ cups skim milk
1 1.4-ounce package sugar-free chocolate pudding mix
8 ounces fat-free whipped topping

Blend cottage cheese, cream cheese, milk, and pudding mix in a food processor (you may need to blend in two batches to avoid overflowing). Fold in whipped topping. Pour into 10 individual parfait glasses. Chill and serve.

**Serves 10**

Nutrition information per serving:
Protein: 8 grams
Carbohydrates: 15 grams
Fat: 0 grams
Calories: 102

# 9

## Real-World Strategies

By this point in your becoming a master of the Link-and-Balance Eating Method, you might be thinking, "I can do link and balance at home, but what happens when I go out?" This section of the book will show you how to handle real-world situations. These include cooking convenient "fast foods" at home and eating at restaurants, whether for fine dining or fast food.

## Link, Balance, and Juggle—Convenience Foods at Home

We know how hard it is to think about linking and balancing when you are already juggling a busy lifestyle. Remember that it will get easier as you develop a pattern that works for you. Eating at home does not have to mean cooking a three-course meal. Convenience foods can be used to make life easier. The following convenience items are already linked, balanced, and low in fat. In other words, they have no more than 38 grams of carbohydrates, at least 14 grams of protein, and no more than 10 grams of fat per serving. Add these to your routine and you'll be able to link, balance, and juggle without missing a beat.

⅛ of a pizza made with 1 16-ounce *Boboli* thin pizza crust
topped with pizza sauce, 16 ounces of fat-free pizza
cheese, fresh vegetables, Canadian bacon, 99 percent fat-
free ham, shrimp, and reduced-fat pepperoni.

1 portion of any *Chef's Choice Stirfries*

1 cup *chili*, any of these brands:

    Hormel 99 percent fat-free chili

    Nalleys 99 percent fat-free chili

    Stagg 99 percent fat-free chili

1 serving of a *frozen dinner*, any of these brands and
varieties:

    Banquet—turkey, mostly white meat

    Budget Gourmet—fettuccine with meatballs in wine sauce or
        glazed turkey

    Healthy Choice—beef peppers Cantonese, chicken Dijon,
        chicken picante, chicken teriyaki, or grilled chicken with
        mashed potatoes

    Lean Cuisine—oven-roasted beef, cheese cannelloni

    Marie Callender's—grilled turkey breast with rice

    Smart Ones—chicken enchilada suiza, garden lasagna, or grilled
        Salisbury

*Great Starts low-fat breakfast muffin*

1 cup of *Hamburger Helper* made with 1 pound of leanest
ground beef and deleting butter, margarine, and oil, any
of the following varieties:

    barbecue beef, beef stew, beef pasta, cheddar cheese melt,
        cheesy Italian, chili macaroni, Italian herb, pizza pasta,
        potato stroganoff, ravioli, Salisbury, southwest beef,
        stroganoff, zesty Italian

1 serving of *Lean Pockets*, all varieties

½ cup *pasta sauce* with 1 cup pasta and 2 ounces leanest
ground beef, ground turkey breast, 97 percent fat-free
turkey sausage or Italian sausage, shrimp, or vegetarian
meat substitute (1½ cups pasta, sauce, and meat
combined), any of these brands and varieties:

    Classico—mushroom and ripe olive, pecorino Romano and
        herb, roasted garlic, spicy red pepper, or tomato and basil

Del Monte—garlic and onion, traditional, Italian herb, or garlic
herb

Healthy Choice—all varieties

Hunt's—cheese and garlic, four cheese, Italian sausage,
mushroom, roasted garlic, or traditional

Newman's Own—Sockarooni, Venetian, or Venetian with
mushrooms

Prego—diced onion and garlic, garden combination, garlic
supreme, three cheese, or vegetable supreme

Ragu—hearty or light

*5 Ruiz Beef Taquitos*

*Soups,* in these brands, varieties, and amounts:

Anderson's split pea, 1 cup

Campbell's Chunky—beef pasta, 1½ cups; beef potato, 1½
cups; bean and ham, 1 cup; chicken noodle, 2 cups;
hearty chicken, 2 cups; pepper steak, 1½ cups; or split
pea and ham, 1 cup

Campbell's Healthy Request—chicken noodle, 2 cups; split
pea, 1 cup; or vegetable beef, 1½ cups

1 package Fantastic Foods—black bean, cha-cha chili, or
split pea

Healthy Choice—bean and ham, 1 cup; chicken and rice, 2
cups; split pea, 1 cup

1 package Nile Spice—black bean, lentil, or split pea

Progresso—99 percent fat-free beef barley, 1 cup; beef
barley, 1 cup; 99 percent fat-free chicken noodle, 1 cup;
lentil, 1 cup; split pea with ham, 1 cup

Progresso White Meat—chicken and rice, 1 cup; chicken and
rotini, 1 cup; chicken barley, 1 cup; chicken noodle, 1
cup; chicken vegetable, 1 cup; rotisserie seasoned
chicken, 1 cup

*StarKist Charlie's tuna lunch kit*

¾ cup *Suddenly Salad* with 8 ounces cubed 99 percent
fat-free ham, turkey, or chicken breast added and
following the low-fat directions, any flavor

1 cup cheesy pasta *Tuna Helper* made with one 6-ounce can of
water-packed tuna and deleting butter, margarine, and oil

# Fine Dining

The most important thing to remember when you dine out is to enjoy yourself. Enjoy your company, the ambiance, the smells, and the sights all around you. Savor the experience as well as the food itself. If you do happen to overindulge, don't beat yourself up. Think about how you could do things differently next time. Get right back to your link-and-balance plan. If you do this promptly, the small amount of weight you may have gained will come off quickly! This is especially important to remember when you return from a vacation, where dining out occurs more often.

Dining out can be a challenge when you're trying to develop an eating routine. At home you know what to expect, but when you are away from home, it may be difficult to anticipate what you will find. Planning ahead can be helpful. Here are some tips for planning for a meal at a restaurant.

• **Don't skip meals before you go out.** This will make you hungrier, which may cause you to overeat. You may also prime your body to store fat by putting yourself into a fasting state. Eat as you normally would prior to going out. In fact, you may want to have a snack prior to going out if you anticipate that you may be eating later than usual. If you do eat more than you should while dining out, doing some physical activity afterward may help you to burn those extra calories. (See Chapter 10 for more information on activities for burning fat.)

• **Before going out, decide if you will be including any splurges.** Splurges are important to include on a routine basis in order to meet your emotional needs. However, splurging is to be done in moderation. If you eat out for 90 percent of your meals, it would not be appropriate to include a splurge each time. It is important to allow yourself a splurge for special events, such as a piece of cake on your birthday or an indulgence on your anniversary. If you are going to have a high-carbohydrate food such as a sweet dessert, you may want to have little or no other high-carbohydrate foods at the meal—and be sure to link with protein.

• **Be wary of sauces, salad dressings, condiments on sandwiches, butter on bread, and toppings for potatoes.** Ask about these things when you place your order so that there will be no surprises. Restaurant foods are usually higher in fat than what you eat at home. Ask

> *You can lose any weight that you gain in one-third of the time it took you to gain it—if you get right back to your plan.*

the server what menu items she or he would suggest that are low in fat. Your server can ask the chef to substitute lower-fat ingredients when possible.

• **If you are ordering a salad or fixing yourself one at a salad bar, use reduced-fat or fat-free dressings if they are available.** If they are not available, consider having lemon juice or vinegar with very little oil or simply ask for the dressing on the side and use very little of it. Remember that each tablespoon of regular salad dressing provides about one hundred calories. It is not unusual for a salad at a restaurant to be topped with four hundred calories' worth of dressing alone! Olives, bacon bits, sunflower seeds, oil-marinated artichoke hearts, and other items can raise the calorie count to almost 1,000. If you are having salad as a main course, be sure to have one with protein, such as grilled chicken salad or shrimp salad.

• **If you are served portions that are too large, stop eating when you have had enough and ask the server to put the rest in a take-out container.** Do this as soon as possible so you won't be tempted to nibble as you socialize. If you know that portions will be large and that you will have a hard time resisting overeating, consider ordering from the appetizer menu or splitting a meal with your dinnermate or ordering a child's or senior's portion.

• **If you have a choice between a baked potato, rice pilaf, French fries, or mashed potatoes, decide which will best help you to meet your goals.** A baked potato is low in fat and can be a good choice but is definitely a splurge if you know you will want sour cream, butter, and bacon bits on it. Rice pilaf is usually a low-fat choice. French fries are very high in fat and calories. Restaurant mashed potatoes are usually made with butter and possibly other high-fat additives. Ask your server to substitute two nonstarchy vegetables instead.

• **Decide if wine or other alcoholic beverages are important to you.** They are splurges. Keep in mind that they do add extra calories, especially if sweet mixers are added. They also have an appetite-stimulating effect, so you may end up eating more than you planned. Alcohol also slows down metabolism, and therefore you may not lose weight for several days following such a splurge. This is why we recommend keeping alcohol intake to two drinks a week for weight loss.

• **Refresh and refocus yourself prior to going out with a few minutes to reflect on your vision and goals. Use positive self-talk to support your weight goal.** This will relax you, feed your emotional needs, and make it easier for you to enjoy your meal without overindulging.

## Tips for Choosing Menu Items at Specific Types of Restaurants

### Steak Houses

A sirloin steak is a good choice. You may find that all chicken and fish options are breaded and deep-fried, so ask if you are not sure. Remember the tips mentioned earlier in regard to salad bars. Watch the portion on a baked potato; they are often huge. And remember to tell the server what you would like on it. Butter *and* sour cream are usually not necessary. (Chives and salt and pepper are fat-free and calorie-free!)

### Chinese Restaurants

Asian food is often low in fat and calories. Be wary of deep-fried items, such as prawns, almond chicken, and sweet-and-sour pork. These are *not* low in fat or calories. Sweet-and-sour sauces are also very high in carbohydrates. Stir-fries, broth-based soups, chow mein, chop suey, and egg foo yung are all good choices. Watch the amount of rice and noodles that you eat; limit these carbohydrate foods to about two-thirds cup total.

### Italian Restaurants

Don't be afraid of pasta or pizza! Just watch the amount that you eat and be sure to link with protein. One cup of pasta is two high-carbohydrate servings. One and a half pieces of thin-crust pizza (medium-sized) is also equal to two servings of carbohydrates. Bread and breadsticks would add even more carbohydrates, and the garlic butter or olive oil adds fat. Pepperoni, sausage, and olives are also high in fat. Canadian bacon or ham, pineapple, vegetables other than olives, or just plain cheese pizza are all lower-fat topping options.

### Mexican Restaurants

Many Mexican restaurant menu items are low in fat. Watch out for those that are deep-fried, like chimichangas, tortilla chips, nachos, crisp burritos, and Mexi-fries. Corn and soft tortillas, or hard taco shells are better low-fat options. Guacamole and sour cream also add fat, but salsa is fat-free usually. Beans are a good source of protein. Be aware that veggie burritos are often too high in carbohydrates because of the large tortilla and the rice.

### Fish Houses

More restaurants are now offering lower-fat fish options in addition to the high-fat deep-fried choices. Ask if the baked fish is made with a butter sauce. Sautéed, steamed, or poached fish is usually low in fat. Again, consider side dish options. But the standard fries are not low in fat! Coleslaw and clam chowder probably are not either.

### Breakfast and Pancake Houses

One pancake with two tablespoons of syrup and two eggs is a perfect balance. Two eggs prepared any way with one or two pieces of toast will also balance. Sausage and bacon do not count as protein. They are almost pure fat. But a ham slice is a good protein source. Hashed brown potatoes are usually loaded with fat.

### Buffets

All-you-can-eat buffets can be good in some ways and difficult in other ways. Buffets usually have many high-protein choices, which may or may not be low in fat. Although prime rib is very high in fat, other roasts are lower. Ham roasts typically are not low in fat. Steamed vegetables are often available and are an excellent choice. It is usually possible to find choices that will fit your eating plan. However, the availability of so many choices may also make it difficult for you. If you know that you will overeat to "get your money's worth" at all-you-can-eat buffets, you may want to avoid going to them. If you can adhere to your plan without this being a problem, then buffets may be a great choice.

# Fast-Food and Chain Restaurants

The fast-food choices that follow are all linked and balanced and are low-fat choices. When you are in a hurry, think of these options at the drive-through window. Any one of these choices has 35 grams of carbohydrates or less, 14 grams of protein or more, and 15 grams of fat or less. They're the perfect combination for when you are on the run. These choices are without mayonnaise or sauces unless listed otherwise, so be sure to request that when ordering. Optional items apply to all choices that precede them.

### Arby's

light roast chicken deluxe
light roast turkey deluxe
light roast beef deluxe
junior roast beef sandwich
grilled chicken barbecue minus ¼ of the bun
ham and cheese
ham and cheese melt
roast chicken salad with croutons and fat-free dressing
chef salad with croutons and fat-free dressing
Timberline chili
Boston clam chowder or cream of broccoli soup and 8 ounces
    of 2% milk
Optional: a side salad with reduced-calorie Italian dressing
    minus croutons, Arby's sauce, au jus, light cholesterol-free
    mayonnaise, ketchup, and mustard

### Big Boy

turkey sandwich
chicken with mozzarella sandwich
chicken breast dinner with bread and salad with buttermilk
    dressing

chicken breast dinner with mozzarella with bread and salad
with buttermilk dressing
Cajun cod dinner with bread and salad with buttermilk
dressing
baked or broiled cod minus Dijon with bread and salad with
buttermilk dressing
Cajun dinner with bread and salad with buttermilk dressing
Dijon chicken breast salad
Optional: cabbage soup, green beans, carrots, or mixed
vegetables

### Blimpie

grilled chicken salad with vinegar minus salad dressing
6-inch Blimpie Best, club, grilled chicken, ham and Swiss,
roast beef, or turkey sub sandwich with no mayonnaise
minus ⅔ of the bread

### Bojangles

Cajun roast chicken without skin
chicken bites
Optional: green beans and Cajun pintos, marinated coleslaw,
or potatoes minus gravy

### Burger King

chef salad with croutons and fat-free dressing
chicken salad with croutons and fat-free dressing
BK Broiler chicken sandwich without mayonnaise and a side
salad with croutons and fat-free dressing
hamburger
Optional: garden salad or side salad with reduced-calorie
light Italian dressing and lettuce, tomato, onion, pickles,
ketchup, and mustard

### Carl's Junior

junior hamburger
barbecue charbroiled chicken
charbroiled chicken salad with 2 breadsticks

Optional: garden salad with fat-free Italian dressing
and salsa

## Chick-Fil-A

chicken sandwich
chicken deluxe sandwich
chargrilled chicken sandwich minus ¼ of bun
chargrilled chicken deluxe sandwich minus ¼ of bun
chargrilled chicken club sandwich minus dressing and minus
    ¼ of bun
Chick-n-Q sandwich minus ¼ of bun
chicken salad on whole wheat minus ¼ of bread
chicken strips salad
8 Chick-Fil-A nuggets
Any two of the following items: hearty breast of chicken
    soup, 4 chicken strips, and chargrilled chicken garden
    salad

## Church's Fried Chicken

breast with corn on the cob or potatoes and gravy
3 tender strips with potatoes and gravy

## Dairy Queen

DQ homestyle hamburger
grilled chicken breast fillet sandwich

## Denny's

2 Sunny Fresh egg substitutes or 3 ounces of ham and
    applesauce, ½ plain bagel, 8 ounces oatmeal, 1 plain
    English muffin, 2 slices plain toast, 4 ounces grits
½ grilled chicken sandwich
½ Charleston chicken sandwich
½ Denny burger
garden chicken delite
grilled Alaska salmon or pot roast and mashed potatoes with
    gravy

grilled chicken breast and broccoli in butter sauce, carrots in
   honey glaze, corn in butter sauce, cornbread stuffing,
   green beans with bacon, mashed potatoes and gravy, or
   rice pilaf
junior burger without fries

## Domino's

14- or 12-inch hand-tossed pizza topped with ham and extra
   cheese—1½ slices
⅕ of 14-inch thin-crust ham pizza
1 slice or ¼ of 12-inch thin-crust ham pizza
Optional: green peppers, onions, mushrooms, and banana
   peppers
7 hot wings or barbecue wings and 1 breadstick or 1 piece of
   cheesy bread
Optional: garden salad with light Italian dressing

## Godfather's Pizza

⅙ of small original crust combo pizza
⅕ of small golden crust combo pizza
⅐ of medium-sized golden crust combo pizza
⅒ of large golden crust combo pizza

## Golden Corral

grilled chicken
sirloin steak
steak tips with onions
Optional: ½ baked potato

## Hardee's

hamburger
cheeseburger
grilled chicken sandwich minus ⅛ of bun
hot ham and cheese
Optional: side salad minus dressing or grilled chicken salad
   minus dressing

### Jack in the Box

Breakfast Jack
cheeseburger
chicken fajita pita
4 chicken strips
Optional: side salad with low-calorie Italian dressing or
   garden chicken salad with 2 packages of croutons and
   low-calorie Italian dressing

### Kenny Roger's Roasters

white meat chicken minus skin or sliced turkey breast and a
   side salad with 1 teaspoon dressing, steamed vegetables,
   or tomato-cucumber salad and corn muffin, corn on the
   cob, sweet corn niblets, creamy Parmesan spinach, honey
   baked beans, Italian green beans, macaroni and cheese, or
   zucchini and squash Santa Fe
chicken Caesar salad with 1 teaspoon dressing
roasted chicken salad

### KFC

Tender Roast breast chicken minus skin and corn on the cob
   or a buttermilk biscuit
Tender Roast breast chicken minus skin and green beans or
   Mean Greens, barbecue baked beans, coleslaw, garden
   rice, macaroni and cheese, mashed potatoes with gravy,
   or red beans and rice
barbecue-flavored chicken sandwich

### Little Caesars

½ Baby Pan!Pan! pizza and tossed salad with Italian fat-free
   dressing

### Long John Silver's

1 piece of Flavorbaked fish or chicken or 1 piece of battered
   chicken and cheese sticks, 1 hush puppy, corn cobbette,

rice pilaf, coleslaw, or ocean chef salad with 1 teaspoon
of dressing
popcorn chicken
Flavorbaked fish sandwich
Flavorbaked chicken sandwich
Optional: side salad minus dressing, green beans, ketchup,
shrimp sauce, tartar sauce, honey mustard sauce, malt
vinegar, or sweet-and-sour sauce

## McDonald's

grilled chicken salad deluxe with croutons and fat-free
dressing
grilled chicken deluxe sandwich minus ¼ of bun
cheeseburger
hamburger and 1% milk
4 Chicken McNuggets and 1% milk
Optional: garden salad with ½ package of fat-free herb
dressing
egg McMuffin
English muffin with 2 scrambled eggs

## Perkins

Denver omelet with fruit cup
seafood omelet with fruit cup
½ pita stir-fry
mini chef salad with 8 saltines

## Pizza Hut

1½ slices Thin 'n Crispy cheese, beef, ham, or pepperoni pizza
1¼ slices Thin 'n Crispy Italian sausage, pork, supreme, or
super supreme; hand-tossed cheese, beef, ham, pepperoni,
Italian sausage, or pork; pan cheese, beef, ham,
pepperoni, or pork pizza
1 slice Thin 'n Crispy Meat Lover's; hand-tossed Meat
Lover's, Pepperoni Lover's, supreme, or super supreme;
pan Pepperoni Lover's, supreme, or super supreme pizza

### Red Lobster

catfish, mackerel, Norwegian salmon, or rainbow trout, lunch
portion, prepared with no added fat
Atlantic cod, flounder, grouper, haddock, halibut, lemon
sole, monkfish, Atlantic perch, pollack, red rockfish,
red snapper, sockeye salmon, swordfish, tilefish, or
yellowfin tuna, lunch or dinner portion, prepared with
no added fat
16 ounces king crab legs
16 ounces snow crab legs
5 ounces langoustine
18 ounces Maine lobster
13 ounces rock lobster
5 ounces calico scallops
5 ounces deep sea scallops
7 ounces shrimp
8 ounces sirloin steak
4 ounces skinless chicken breast

### Round Table Pizza

⅛ of Alfredo Contempo, chicken and garlic gourmet, or
Western barbecue supreme thin-crust pizza
1¼ slices Alfredo Contempo pan pizza
1¾ slices zesty Santa Fe chicken thin-crust pizza

### Shoney's

baked fish with ½ baked potato
½ charbroiled chicken sandwich
½ chicken fillet sandwich
light fried fish
Hawaiian chicken
½ seafood platter
½ charbroiled steak and shrimp
½ Italian feast

## Skipper's

3 "Lite Catch" chicken tenderloin strips
3 chicken strips
baked salmon with ½ baked potato
smoked salmon chowder or clam chowder with 2 chicken
    strips or shrimp and seafood salad with low-calorie
    Italian dressing or 1 teaspoon of other dressing
Optional: side salad with low-calorie Italian dressing

## Sizzler

lemon herb chicken breast
Santa Fe chicken breast
broiled shrimp
shrimp scampi
Optional: baked potato minus skin or 4 ounces broccoli
    cheese soup with 2 saltines, 6 ounces clam chowder,
    3 pieces focaccia bread, 2 ounces pasta with 3 meatballs,
    2 ounces potato skins, taco shell with 2 ounces taco
    filling and ¼ cup refried beans, ¼ cup carrot and raisin
    salad, 2 cups Chinese chicken salad, 2 cups Mediter-
    ranean minted fruit, ½ cup Mexican fiesta salad,
    ½ cup old-fashioned potato salad, ¼ cup red herb
    potato salad, ½ cup seafood Louis pasta salad, ¾ cup
    seafood salad, 1 cup teriyaki beef salad, ¼ cup tuna
    pasta, ½ cup peaches, or ½ cup chocolate or vanilla
    soft-serve dessert
hibachi chicken breast with pineapple
4 fried shrimp
3 to 4 ounces Dakota ranch steak
salmon
swordfish
Optional: 4 ounces chicken noodle or minestrone soup, 2
    ounces spicy jicama salad, or green salad with ¼ cup
    cottage cheese, lite Italian dressing, and Japanese rice
    vinegar

### Subway

6-inch club, steak and cheese, roast beef, turkey breast, or
ham and cheese sub without mayonnaise or oil
Optional: mustard, ketchup, vinegar, salt, pepper, and all
vegetables except olives

### Taco Bell

pintos and cheese minus sour cream
chicken fajita minus sour cream
chicken soft taco minus sour cream

### Wendy's

grilled chicken sandwich minus mayonnaise
junior hamburger with ketchup and mustard
grilled chicken salad with fat-free dressing and croutons
Wendy's chili

# 10

# Fitness Matters

Physical activity can greatly speed up your weight-loss program and is essential for maintaining your desired weight and your general health. There are at least four main ways that activity helps your body:

1. Increased physical activity has been found to lower insulin resistance by making the muscle fibers use glucose more efficiently.

2. Physically, the calorie-burning and metabolism-increasing effects of activity speed up fat loss and improve muscle tone.

3. Physical activity increases the amount of mood enhancers called *endorphins* in your brain. Endorphins contribute to your feelings of well-being.

4. Emotionally, the time spent doing the activity is internally registered as valuable "self time." This enhances your sense of self-nurturing, the most powerful of all maintenance promoters. When you continue an activity program, you sustain self-nurturing.

The three types of fat-burning exercise are

- Brisk activity
- Aerobic activity
- Muscle-building activity

> *Regular physical activity is another key to success in your weight control.*

# Brisk Activity

Brisk activity should not be too strenuous when you want maximum fat burning and weight loss. Walking, gardening, or housecleaning can be very effective. Other good brisk activities include swimming, cross-country skiing, or rowing, as long as you do them at a moderate pace. Brisk activity differs from aerobic activity in that it does not increase your heart rate to a training rate. It is simply moving your arms and legs. Brisk activity is the most effective activity for fat burning. Brisk activity does not have to be continuous to burn fat. In fact, intermittent activity, such as climbing stairs several times each day or walking a few blocks to and from your car, also helps. Studies have shown that even activity such as jiggling your leg while sitting increases fat burning. So don't just sit there; do something as you sit. Stand up and walk around a bit when you're on the phone. Work in activity of any kind as often as you can.

# Aerobic Activity

Aerobic activity increases your metabolic rate so you will burn more calories throughout the day. *Metabolic rate* is the speed at which you use up energy. This rate will remain increased for the entire day and into the next day, having a sustained effect for thirty-six hours. Aerobic activity helps your body use carbohydrates more efficiently.

But more aerobic activity is not better. Researchers have found that only twelve minutes a day of aerobic activity for six days a week or twenty-five minutes for three days a week is enough to increase your metabolic rate. Don't do more than twenty-five minutes of aerobic activity at a time. It is not necessary, and contrary to popular belief, it may actually slow down or stop your weight loss. This is because the fast pace of aerobic activity demands a large amount of glucose. Your body will start by using any carbohydrates that you have recently eaten. Then it uses up "emergency" sources of stored glucose, called *glycogen*, from the muscles and liver. After these glucose stores are used up, which usually happens within the first twenty-five minutes of aerobic activity, you will start to break down muscle. The amount of muscle mass that you carry sets your metabolic rate. Less muscle leads to a slower metabolism, which means less weight loss. If you build up to an aggressive activity program, be sure to eat enough protein. Otherwise you will lose muscle mass. Only protein can make muscle, and muscle must be made every day.

Your body cannot burn fat during aerobic activity. Changing fat into glucose for body energy is a very complex and slow process. Your body cannot burn fat under the high glucose demands of aerobic activity. If your goal is fat loss, it is better to stop aerobic activity after twenty-five minutes and add in some muscle-building or brisk activity if you want to continue exercising. When we perform body composition tests on our patients, we see muscle mass actually decrease over time in people who do too much aerobic activity. This can be good for a marathon runner who wants long, lean, strong muscles but not for a person who is trying to lose weight. (*Body composition tests* measure the amounts of fat and muscle on the body.) So remember that activity is a good thing, but you can do *too much* of a good thing.

Aerobic activity includes moderate exercise that will increase your heart rate but still allow you to carry on a conversation. Consult an aerobic trainer for information on how to determine your optimal target heart rate during exercise or see the sidebar on the next page.

## Muscle-Building Activity

Muscle-building activity increases the amount of muscle on your body. Having more muscle increases your metabolic rate. Muscle-building activity involves exercises that use resistance in pulling, pushing, or lifting.

Some easy ways to increase muscle mass using resistance are as follows:

- Add light hand or ankle weights when you walk. One- or two-pound weights are a good choice. Be careful not to swing your arms too much, which would cause you to throw yourself off balance.

*5–10 minutes of warm-up*

*20–25 minutes of aerobic activity with your pulse at your target heart rate*

*To calculate your target pulse, subtract your age from 220, and then multiply that number by 0.75. The answer is the number of beats per minute you should feel when you take your pulse.*

*For example: 220 minus 45 (years old) is 175. Then 0.75 × 175 equals 131. So 131 beats per minute is the optimal pulse rate during this phase of aerobic activity.*

*15–20 minutes of cool-down*

Keep your arms close to your chest, and pump them up and down. Think about wearing your light ankle weights around the house or yard while you are doing chores. You might even strap them on at work, concealed under pants, making muscle while you work!

• Use the force of gravity against your body for resistance by doing leg lifts, sit-ups, or pull-ups. Working the larger muscles in your legs will increase your total muscle mass the fastest. Sit-ups may firm your stomach but will not increase muscle mass quickly. Using ankle weights or resistance "rubber bands" during leg lifts will give you even greater resistance.

• Do lunges as you talk on the phone.

• Lift up on your toes while you are standing at work, while doing dishes, or while folding clothes.

It is best not to work the same muscles two days in a row because muscles need time to recover. So work your legs one day and your upper body the next. About ten minutes each day is ideal. Or do aerobics one day and muscle building the next. You can develop your own plan.

# Exercise Advice

You may wish to monitor your weight loss by following your body-fat-to-muscle ratio. Fitness clubs and some physicians have body composition analysis machines that easily and accurately tell you how effective your fitness program is.

You want to avoid muscle wasting (sarcopenia), which occurs when you lose weight too fast or in any other unhealthy manner. Less muscle results in a slowed metabolism and a tendency to regain weight more rapidly. Usually the weight regained is a higher percentage of fat than before.

The most important thing about any activity plan is that it is enjoyable and fits into your lifestyle. Adoption of a lifetime activity habit is the key to weight maintenance. This has been the conclusion of every study done on weight-loss maintenance. All people who fell off their activity program gained their weight back within two years, most gaining more weight than they had lost! Only those who continued their activity program were able to successfully keep their weight off for the long term.

Selection of likeable and doable activity is the key to sustaining a lifetime pattern of activity. Don't do jumping jacks or sit-ups if you hate doing them. Find some activities that you enjoy. To break the boredom, alternate several of them. And don't think that you have to take an hour to change into workout clothes and go to the gym. There are many activities that you can do on your fifteen-minute break at work or in your own living room while you are watching your favorite television shows. In fact, watching TV or socializing with friends as you do your activity will help the time seem shorter.

## *Getting Rid of Fat Around the Waist*

There is no direct way to get rid of fat in any particular area of the body. Even doing a lot of sit-ups or abdominal crunches will simply firm the underlying stomach muscles. It will not budge the overlying fat. The best way to trim your waist is to activate your larger muscle groups such as the thigh and buttock muscles. Working these muscles increases your body's overall metabolism and speeds up fat burning.

## *Eating and Exercise*

Since only carbohydrates can give you immediate energy, it is important to eat some carbohydrates right before your workout. Remember to link them with a protein. Yogurt with fruit is a good linked choice. Crackers and cheese will also energize your workout.

Working out first thing in the morning or right after work without eating significantly reduces the effectiveness of your activity. In this case, you are wasting valuable effort without the help of carbohydrate energy. Your performance and endurance really suffer. Your body starts stealing from your muscles in order to find the energy to make it through your workout. You most likely will lose muscle weight rather than unwanted fat weight.

# Your Fitness Action Plan

When you plan your activity, remember this advice:

- Do it with someone else.
- Do it with something else, like handheld weights, elastic bands, or an exercise ball.
- Do it with enjoyment. Do only the activities that you like.

The ideal fitness action plan includes these three phases:

1. As much brisk (nonaerobic) activity as possible

2. Twenty-five minutes of aerobic activity three times a week

3. Ten minutes each day or twenty minutes every other day of muscle-building activity.

Right now, while you are thinking about it, list five activities that you can start on right away. Choose one and start doing it. We recommend exercising in the morning after a light snack. This way, the task is already done for the day. Add more activity as you are able until you have included some of each of the three types of activity: brisk, aerobic, and muscle-building. Remember not to overdo the aerobic activity!

*Medical precautions: Before starting any exercise program always check with your doctor! This is especially true if you have ever had high blood pressure, heart rhythm irregularities, a heart attack, a stroke, or diabetes. Your doctor may prescribe special tests to assess your body's ability to undergo strenuous physical activity.*

# 11

# Appetite vs. Hunger

## *Understanding Our Relationship with Food*

**W**hile the Insulin-Resistance Diet program and most other weight-loss plans focus on the types and amounts of food you eat, we know from our experiences and those of our patients that maintenance of weight has very little to do with food. Successful weight maintenance has more to do with realizing, expressing, and satisfying our deep internal needs. Achieving this goal gives you a sense of control over your life that is essential for truly being happy about yourself.

*Hunger* is the actual physical need for food to sustain your body. It is normal for the body to be hungry every three to five hours. If you feel hungry before this interval, your diet may be deficient in protein.

*Appetite*, on the other hand, represents the emotional needs you have that must be met. Overeating is often an indication that emotional needs are not being met. This is especially true when you can't put the words *control* and *your life* in the same sentence. Unmet needs may not be obvious. They may be hiding in your subconscious and may be somewhat immediate or may have developed when you were a very small child.

It is important that you listen to your body's hunger signals. If you feel hungry, then you should have something to eat. Don't make yourself wait until the next meal. Being overly hungry by that mealtime will cause you to overeat.

It is also very important that you do not ignore your appetite, your emotional food needs. All people need some emotional involvement with food. This is one of the reasons why humans were blessed with the senses of smell and taste. It is human nature to explore and enjoy culinary experiences. All "lifetime dieters" tend to try to deny and hide these basic needs, convincing themselves that they must eat to live only. This thinking will lead to yo-yo dieting or binge eating after weight loss. Linking and balancing is not a diet but a lifetime eating method within which you may "feed" your emotional needs often. This means, among other things, allowing yourself to enjoy food again by making time to sit down and relax while eating rather than rushing through a quick bite or eating a candy bar in the closet.

## Action Plan

Get started on your own investigation by becoming aware of your emotional needs in relation to food; for example, note when you eat and what triggers your appetite (watching TV, being stressed, being bored, etc.). Learn to listen to your body's food needs and answer them. If you still find yourself feeling like you have to eat and you really should not be hungry, stop and think about what is going on around you and how you feel emotionally. Actually write down your observations. If you do this routinely, you will start to see a pattern that you can then correct. Recognizing and transferring stress or boredom eating to more constructive behaviors are essential to successful long-term weight maintenance.

Record the times over the next three days when you feel you really want to eat but you know that you should not be hungry. Remember that it is normal to feel hungry if you have not eaten in the past two or three hours. In that case, you really are hungry and should have a snack. Note how you are feeling at the time and any appetite triggers you may recognize. Next to that, think of an action you can take next time to avoid raiding the fridge.

**Day 1**

_____
_____
_____
_____
_____
_____
_____
_____
_____

**Day 2**

_____
_____
_____
_____
_____
_____
_____
_____

**Day 3**

_____
_____
_____
_____
_____
_____
_____

## Your Relationship with Food: A Self-Test

Food is more than just your fuel. Your relationship with food is unique, personal, and often deeply rooted from childhood. Some people love to plan, shop for, and cook meals while others prefer to deal with food as little as possible. Either situation is OK. It is when you try to fight *against* your food relationship that you create problems. For example, a person who loves to cook but tries to "stay out of the kitchen" while trying to lose weight will not be successful in the long run. It is important to recognize not only that you have this relationship with food but also that you must act on behalf of it if you are to maintain your weight loss long term. We call these ties to food your *food interactive needs*. Food interactive needs may also influence the types of foods you enjoy, such as crunchy versus creamy, or hot versus cold. Try to identify your needs by answering the following list of questions honestly. There are no right or wrong answers.

1. How many times during the day are you face-to-face with food? Three times or fewer? Four to eight times a day? Eight or more times a day?

2. Do you prepare most of the meals for yourself or family?

3. Do you work around food all day, as in a restaurant or bakery?

4. Do you like to have a sweet treat at the end of your day, middle of the day, or all day long?

5. How long do you spend with food? Less than three hours in a day? Three to six hours in a day? More than six hours in a day?

6. Do you have a quick cup of coffee in the morning and then fly out the door?

7. Do you mosey about in the morning, reading the paper and having a leisurely breakfast?

8. Do you have lunch with a friend, chatting and eating for an hour or so?

9. Do you enjoy preparing gourmet meals for your family or friends, spending hours in the kitchen developing your masterpiece?

10. Do you love to read recipes and cookbooks?

11. Do you love to try new recipes?

12. Do you enjoy going to the grocery store and looking over all the new food products?

13. Do you enjoy browsing at a gourmet food store?

14. Do you love kitchen food gadgets?

15. Do you enjoy a morning breakfast ritual?

16. Do you like to chew gum or sip on coffee or soda during the day?

17. Which best describes your preferred meal pattern: three meals a day and no snacks, three meals and at least three snacks, or grazing all day?

18. What textures of foods do you prefer? Crunchy or creamy foods? Wet or dry foods? Hot or cold foods?

Once you realize what some of your food interactive needs are, make an effort to fulfill them when you eat. When you deny, ignore, or are unaware of these needs by eating types of foods or eating at times or in patterns that do not meet your interactive needs, you will have a hard time emotionally registering that you even ate anything. This is one of the most important areas that we have worked on with our patients for their long-term success.

The interaction you have with food all really happens before you even swallow. Once you swallow, your interaction with food is over. So focus on everything important to you about that food before swallowing it. This is like the fine art of wine tasting. Much of the time overeating occurs simply because you ate foods that didn't register as satisfying to you. Maybe you ate tons of creamy, soft foods, but what you really wanted was something crunchy and salty. Learn to recognize your food needs so that you can answer them right away.

## Rating Your Food Choices

On a scale of one to ten, with ten being your best choice, rate your typical food choices. Then try to eat foods you rate as seven or better as often as you can. At least half of the food you eat during the day should be rated this high. Of course, you rank certain foods higher at certain times and lower at other times. Sometimes an apple will rate a three for you and sometimes it will be a ten.

Over the next three days, keep a food log. Rate the foods you eat on this scale. Be sure to rate these choices according to how you feel about them before you eat them.

**Day 1**

_____

_____

_____

_____

_____

_____

_____

_____

**Day 2**

_____

_____

_____

_____

_____

_____

_____

_____

**Day 3**

_____

_____

_____

_____

_____

_____

_____

_____

# Splurging . . . Yes!

**Sharon**—*Sharon told us the first time that she visited our clinic that she had gone on her first diet at the age of eight. Since that time she has tried every diet she could find. Only a few of them were successful and each time success was only temporary. After each success she returned to her old ways of eating and regained all of her weight and sometimes even more. It was not possible to eat only "diet foods" for the rest of her life.*

*Sharon was very excited to try a program that did not require counting calories or fat grams or require cutting out all of her favorite foods. She was pleased that she did not have to starve herself, too. She was a little apprehensive as to whether or not the Insulin-Resistance Diet would work for her. Her second visit to the Wellness Workshop assured her that she would lose weight. In fact, she lost nine pounds in two weeks. But she was still afraid to eat many of her favorite foods, and she was eating far too few calories. Several visits later she was eating a very healthy diet, including plenty of calories, but still was eating only "diet foods." She had not eaten any of the foods she loved in weeks. She was getting bored and frustrated despite a steady weight loss. Her "dieting" path was heading for disaster—again.*

*We finally convinced Sharon to eat some of her favorite foods while still adhering to our program. When she arrived for her next appointment, she said, "I know I've gained weight." She was concerned because she had included a small bowl of chocolate ice cream in her plan. To her amazement and delight she did lose weight at the same rate that she had been. Now she was ready to commit to a new way of eating—for a lifetime. Several years later, she continues to maintain a healthy weight, for the first time in her life.*

You understand that some foods are good for your physical needs and others are not as good, especially those that are high in sugar and fat, such as Sharon's bowl of ice cream. However, it is not realistic or even healthy to try to avoid these foods for the rest of your life. Understand that there are no "bad" foods; some foods are simply more important for your emotional health than your physical health. Eat these foods on an occasional basis. We call this *splurging*.

Splurging is critical to your weight-loss and weight-maintenance success. Once you realize the importance of splurging, you will be able to free yourself from the guilt that you may have felt in the past. Many people respond to this guilt by overeating high-fat, high-sugar foods for a while afterward because they feel that they have already blown their diets.

Uncontrollable overeating is called *binge eating*. This can result from being too deprived during weight-loss efforts. Splurging is the controlled form of enjoying foods that you really miss. Eating these foods in a controlled way is a skill to be practiced. Follow these few simple guidelines to enjoy splurging:

• Go ahead and splurge when you feel that it is important for your emotional needs. This is especially important when you are at a party.

• Any type of food can be considered your splurge, as long as you think of it as special at the time.

• When you do splurge, sit down and enjoy your food. Perhaps eat it on your good china with a fancy napkin. Or enjoy your favorite food in a bubble bath. When you are feeding your emotional needs, everything around the food counts, not just the food itself. Emotional needs are met by everything that happens before you swallow the food: anticipating, planning, preparing, seeing, smelling, and tasting. Make all of these things really count!

• Remember that if your splurge is a high-sugar food, watch the amount that you eat and remember to link and balance it with a high-protein food.

## Splurging Action Plan

Practice splurging once a day for the next three days. Write down your splurge along with the food you used to link and balance your splurge. You'll see that by practicing and expecting your splurges you will continue to be in good control of your food choices. Now, regularly splurge at least two days per week. Get in the habit of healthy splurging.

**Day 1**

_____

_____

_____

_____

_____

_____

_____

_____

**Day 2**

_____

_____

_____

_____

_____

_____

_____

**Day 3**

_____

_____

_____

_____

_____

_____

_____

_____

# Hunger Is All in Your Head

All of your hunger signals come from the brain and are under the control of strong messengers called *neurotransmitters*. Over fifty different types of these biochemical messengers carry signals around the brain. Some neurotransmitters help you with energy while others help you to relax or to sleep. Some allow you to laugh, while others let you feel sadness. Neurotransmitters are needed to help you think and to concentrate. In fact, neurotransmitters are needed for about everything you physically and mentally do. A few of the more commonly known neurotransmitters include *melatonin*, which helps you to sleep, *endorphins*, which give you feelings of well-being, and *dopamine* and *serotonin*, which are the masters of your appetite.

## Dopamine and Serotonin

Dopamine and serotonin are the most important neurotransmitters for appetite control. Even though you feel an abdominal stretching discomfort when you overstuff your stomach, the message of feeling full really is all in your head in the form of dopamine and serotonin levels. These neurotransmitters tell you when you are hungry, what you are hungry for, and when you are full enough. High levels of these messengers satisfy your appetite, while low levels cause you to become hungry or to overeat.

Cravings for caffeine, chocolate, sweets, fried foods, or salty foods indicate low or depleted dopamine levels, while cravings for breads and pasta signal low serotonin levels. These important appetite transmitters can be drained to low levels if you are under physical or emotional stress. Lack of enough sleep, restricting important nutrients in your diet, environmental toxins, and taking certain medications can also deplete neurotransmitter amounts. All of these conditions could cause a prolonged chronic shortage of neurotransmitters. Without the adequate messages, your appetite sense would be distorted, leading to overeating or compulsive thoughts about food. Lack of willpower is really a biochemical deficiency of neurotransmitters in the hunger center of the brain. This deficiency occurs especially when you are under a lot of stress.

Some people are genetically unable to make enough of these neurotransmitters. This helps to explain why some eating disorders and weight problems can develop at very young ages.

Dopamine and serotonin also control the emotion center of the brain. This is the center that helps us to cope with conflict, stress, and other feelings. When we are low in or lacking these neurotransmitters we may feel depressed, lethargic, angry, or anxious. Significant emotional illness can result from inadequate levels of these messengers. The more stress you are experiencing, the more neurotransmitters you need for healthy coping. When you are under stress, most of the available dopamine and serotonin neurotransmitters are used up by your brain's emotion center. This then leaves a deficit for controlling the hunger center. This can lead to nervous eating, boredom eating, and loss of food willpower despite your knowing better.

Your levels of dopamine and serotonin change all of the time. They can shift hourly, daily, and monthly depending on your diet, stress level, hormone levels, and physical health. A good example of this flux is that experienced by women with premenstrual syndrome (PMS). As the hormone cycle shifts mid month, the neurotransmitter balance also shifts, and symptoms of irritability, lethargy, food cravings, and anxiety may occur.

Now that scientists have finally been able to identify these neurotransmitters and what they do, they may develop replacement therapies that can help improve people's physical and mental health. At the present time, there are no medications that actually replace the brain's supply of dopamine and serotonin. Your body has to naturally make them from scratch using either the food you eat or dietary supplements you take. Commonly prescribed antidepressant medications, such as Prozac, Paxil, Zoloft, Celexa, Effexor, and Wellbutrin, work by using the dopamine or serotonin already in the brain. These medications do not work very well if you are already depleted of neurotransmitters. This depletion explains why these medication doses may have to be increased to work better.

The right amount of dopamine helps you feel energetic and less hungry. Symptoms of low levels of dopamine can include the following:

- Depression
- Fatigue
- Decreased sex drive
- Increased appetite: feeling hungry a lot of the time
- Cravings for chocolate, caffeine, sweets, fatty foods, and salty foods
- Chronic allergies, headaches, and muscle aches
- Premenstrual breast tenderness

The right amount of serotonin helps you feel calm and secure. Symptoms of low levels of serotonin can include the following:

- Anxiety
- Irritability
- Anger
- Restlessness
- Difficulty knowing when you feel full
- Cravings for bread, bagels, and pasta
- Cravings for alcohol and nicotine
- Premenstrual symptoms of mood and appetite changes
- Psoriasis

## Neurotransmitters and Natural Appetite Regulators

Eating certain foods or adding specific nutrient supplements can increase the levels of dopamine and serotonin in your brain. These nutrients come mainly from protein foods. The protein amino acid tyrosine is needed for dopamine, whereas tryptophan is needed for serotonin. Small amounts of carbohydrates are also necessary to make serotonin. Tyrosine is found mainly in meat and dairy products. Almonds, peanuts, bananas, avocados, lima beans, pickled herring, and pumpkin and sesame seeds also provide amounts of tyrosine. Foods that are highest in tryptophan are turkey and dairy products. Other sources include bananas, dried dates, fish, peanuts, and meat.

Natural nutrient supplements, called *neurotransmitter precursors*, are available at health food stores. These supplements help the brain efficiently manufacture these neurotransmitters without adding a lot of extra calories. These are especially helpful when you're trying to lose weight. Precursors are medically formulated compounds of concentrated amino acids, vitamins, and mineral cofactors. Having adequate amounts of dopamine and serotonin will enable you to have a normal appetite response.

A specialist (physician or naturopath) who has interest and training in *neuroendocrinology*, or natural brain hormone chemistry, would be most helpful in prescribing the right amounts of dopamine and serotonin supplements for you. The commonly prescribed appetite suppressant medications used today work through these dopamine and serotonin pathways. The popular diet pill combination known as Phen-Fen and Redux were medications that controlled appetite through the action of these neurotransmitters. These particular medications are no longer available. As controversial as these medications were, they were successful in restoring a natural, controllable appetite to many patients plagued with overeating because of inadequate amounts of dopamine and serotonin.

Certain activities can also affect the release of more dopamine or serotonin. Rhythmic music with a lot of drums and bass increase dopamine release, while more mellow mood melodies raise serotonin. A warm, relaxing bath can cause a rise in serotonin, so we recommend you try this before your evening meal. The rise in serotonin will make you feel more full, causing you to eat less. An invigorating shower peps up dopamine. Cheering on a winning team, whether on television or in the stadium, releases dopamine. Serotonin soothes your senses when you pet soft, furry animals. Repetitive mouth movements, such as chewing gum, release serotonin, which gives you an increased sense of security. Quiet prayer or meditation also releases serotonin. Tapping your foot, swaying, or dancing to the beat of music is a sure sign that your dopamine has surged. Use these activities to increase or balance out your own dopamine and serotonin levels.

Current research has also identified Neuropeptide Y as the most potent stimulator of appetite yet discovered. Neuropeptide Y starts to rise in the brain within two to three hours after eating. It continues to rise, and once it reaches a critical level, its stimulating power over appetite is virtually impossible to overcome. This helps to explain why it is so difficult to control food choices or portion sizes if you go long periods of time without eating: Neuropeptide Y kicks in and encourages overeating.

Because of continuing medical research, we can see the day in the near future when doctors will be able to pharmacologically supplement low levels of neurotransmitters just as they now directly supplement low hormone levels of thyroid, estrogen, insulin, and cortisone. This therapy will then allow for successful long-term management of some very important emotional and physical health conditions.

# 12

---

# Commitment and Relapse

I f you have made it this far into the Insulin-Resistance Diet program, chances are you are already doing link and balance. If you are, congratulations! Two of the biggest hurdles in accomplishing any worthwhile project or program are providing the commitment to get started and preventing a relapse to your old ways of doing things. In this final chapter we want to motivate you to get going—if you haven't already started on your program—and keep going, until linking and balancing becomes a way of eating that seems natural, working through any relapses that you may occasionally experience.

## If Not Now, When?

### Zeb, Ned, and Zeb's Hound Dog

*Zeb and Ned were sittin' out on the front porch whittlin' wood. Zeb's hound dog was just a-wailin' and a-howlin' and a-whimperin'. Ned says to Zeb, "Zeb, how come yer dog is just a-wailin' and a-howlin' and a-whimperin' over there?"*

*"Oh, he's sittin' on a tack."*

*"Well, how come he don't get off the tack?"*

*"Well, I reckon cause the tack just ain't sharp enough."*

Isn't the idea of this story true for most people? Unless the pain of the experience is bad enough, the misery miserable enough, most people will not make the decision to change. Most people are afraid of change, so they put it off for another day.

The lesson of this story may speak to you as you contemplate weight loss. Did you recently experience a motivating painful event? Did your doctor warn you that you might keel over with a heart attack? Or did you actually have a heart attack? Did you realize that your elevated cholesterol or triglyceride levels are clogging your arteries and are going to shorten your life? Were you recently diagnosed with Type II diabetes? Were you really hurt by an overheard remark about your weight? Were you shocked seeing a recent photograph of yourself? Did you cry in the changing room while trying on clothes?

These are examples of the trigger events that most people experience before real change will occur. The level of commitment required to achieve successful weight loss and then hold onto it is directly related to the amount of pain relief associated with it. We find most of our patients are only truly motivated to begin to lose weight when the pain from being overweight is greater than the pleasure they get from their current lifestyle.

Studies tell us that men are more likely to lose weight for health reasons, such as when they have just had a heart attack. Women tend to take action for self-image reasons. Our own experiences back this up.

When you feel yourself falling away from your intentions, think back to the time of your pain and try to relive it in order to feel the powerful force that propelled you toward a change in the first place. Whether a photograph of the overweight you or a piece of clothing from your larger days, your visit there may bring you to tears. You'll know then that you touched the deepest, most powerful part of yourself.

Finally, taking control of all aspects of your eating challenge may require the help of professionals who keep up with the latest in effective weight-loss management. *Bariatricians*, physicians trained in weight-loss management, are especially sensitive to the struggles you'll encounter while you're trying to lose weight. They are able to apply current medical technology in safe and effective methods. Personal counseling with a therapist may be very helpful for you as you continue on your new journey of healthful change. Keep in mind that improvement in your weight and your health will change the way those closest to you will respond. In order to keep on track with your priorities for your life, communicate openly about this with your family members.

# Your Values and Vision

Right now, sticking with your new lifestyle plan may not seem too difficult. The newness helps keep you focused. The reasons that motivated you to begin this program are fresh in your mind. But as we have said, you may find at some point that your motivation will falter and seem to fade, especially during stressful times. We are not telling you this to discourage you but to make you aware that maintenance of any new lifestyle takes commitment to the values that caused you to begin these lifestyle changes and constant reminders of the vision of what you want to achieve.

## *Values*

What do you value? Is it your health? Is it your looks? Is it your family? Is it your career? Think about the reasons why you wish to change your life through the Insulin-Resistance Diet program. What do you value enough to make these important changes in your life? What goals do you hope to achieve and why? Perhaps you hope for better health to enjoy a longer, healthier life? Or do you desire a more attractive appearance to help your career or social life? Whatever the reasons or values, if they are important to you, they are very important! These are the factors that will motivate you to keep going with your lifestyle changes when things get tough. Take a few moments to actually write down your reasons in a notebook or journal.

## *Vision*

Learn to see your vision. Now that you've identified your goals, close your eyes and envision yourself achieving them. See yourself as the person you have changed into. If you value health, then see yourself playing at the beach or in your backyard with your children or grandchildren—ten, fifteen, even twenty years from now. If appearance is important to you, see yourself going into your clothes closet and picking out beautiful clothes that you will look great in. See yourself going out on a date and feeling confident that you are wonderful and that someone wants to share time with you.

Remember that you design your own vision. List the words you would use to describe yourself in your vision. Use positive descriptive words such as *healthy, strong, vibrant, active, attractive, beautiful, successful, professional, confident.* What descriptive words would you use? Think of as many as you can and write them down in your notebook.

Use these descriptive words often when you are talking to yourself. Positive self-talk will cause positive results. The subconscious part of the brain will do as it is told. If you tell yourself that you are a failure, lazy, and fat and have no self-control, then you will be more of a failure, lazier, and fatter and will have less self-control. But if you remind yourself that you are strong, successful, and in complete control (even if you don't yet feel that way), you will be soon enough. This takes some practicing, though.

You may find it helpful to write your list of positive descriptions on a nice notecard to keep with you or to place somewhere where you will notice it often, such as on your bathroom mirror or in your wallet or day planner. Pictures will help also to remind you of positive thoughts. Look through photo albums for pictures of yourself that remind you of your goal. Or find several realistic pictures from magazines. You may need to rotate your pictures or notecards so that you are more likely to notice them. Make a point to concentrate on these positive images and thoughts several times each day. And most important, if you find yourself using negative self-talk, erase it immediately from your mind and replace it with positive self-talk. The great success motivators of our time, such as Brian Tracy, Anthony Robbins, and Wayne Dyer, all enthusiastically promote the doctrine that whatever you tell yourself that you are is what you will become. Consider getting a book or tape by one of these experts on success and achievement and use him as your personal coach. Your values, visions, and action must all be in alignment for you to meet your goal and maintain it.

# Understanding Relapse

The popular humorist Erma Bombeck commented that she had lost weight so many times that she should be able to fit on a charm bracelet by now. Her story rings true for so many who have had success with weight loss only to regain the weight again and again. This frustrating pattern is called *relapse* and can lead to feelings of shame and guilt.

It is important to accept that relapse is a natural and expected phase that occurs during change. But rather than feeling defeated, use relapse as an opportunity to understand what happened and why. Then you can make appropriate adjustments that will lead you closer to your goals. Letting relapse recur for the same reasons is a definite sign that you need a professional to intervene to help you analyze the less obvious reasons for your actions.

When you relapse, ask yourself this question: why do I do unhealthy things, even though I know better? When you make unhealthy choices, you play one of two roles:

1. **The Victim.** When you consider yourself a victim of an illness, you feel helpless to do much about it. As a victim, you look at the situation with a "Look what it's done to me" attitude.

2. **The Weakling.** The other view is to blame yourself for having such a weak will. With this opposite though equally damaging self-blame, you may tend to be overly hard on yourself, likely wondering, "Why did I do it, for heaven's sake?"

What do you usually say to yourself when you make an unhealthy choice? Both of these unhealthy approaches are paralyzing and will block permanent change. Next time say to yourself, "I can do it!" and keep saying it even if you don't feel it yet. This positive attitude is self-empowering and contagious. Be a winning coach for yourself!

## *Relapse Strategies*

Write at least twenty reasons why you want to lose weight in a notebook or journal. The more reasons you have, the more committed you become to your project. Refer back to this list when you have deviated from the course. You'll find you will recover very quickly.

Acknowledge positive changes that you made with each relapse, no matter how small the change was. Maybe you ate only two boxes of cookies rather than your usual three. Maybe you regained only half of your weight rather than all of it. Maybe you walked around the block once a week rather than not at all. Long-term success is achieved through a process; it is not instantaneous. You need patience in order to accept the normal ups and downs required of positive change. Remember, it's not how far you fall, but how far you bounce.

# Restoring Food Memory

**Maria**—*One of our favorite patients, Maria, who had been a lifelong dieter, told us something very insightful. She told us that the reason she overate was because she had no "food memory." After eating dinner or dessert, she really couldn't remember what her food actually tasted like. So she kept eating and then overeating in order to restore some taste recall. We observed her during several meals and snacks. She read through one of her meals, watched TV during another, and then stood up to eat her snack. It was obvious that she didn't actually lack food memory, but rather she prevented food memory.*

Here are suggestions that have been very helpful to many in restoring food and dining memory. They may not seem quite natural to you now. You need to practice them. They will easily become second nature to you if you intentionally try them for four to six weeks. That is how long it takes any new habit to form.

1. Wait twenty minutes after you eat a meal or snack before eating more. It takes at least twenty minutes after you eat for your food to register in your brain. This is especially important to remember when you still feel hungry after eating. Set a timer if you have to. Feeling full is not an instantaneous signal. The brain does not register stomach fullness until twenty minutes after you have eaten. The average time it takes to eat the food ordered at a fast-food restaurant is seven minutes. Our observations also reveal that overweight people usually eat their meal twice as fast as thinner people. The average sit-down meal at home takes less than ten minutes to eat. A Thanksgiving feast may take hours or days to prepare and

yet only minutes to gobble up. And we wonder why we are always so stuffed after thirty minutes.

2. Try the "three bites of bliss" technique. This is a great exercise. Go out of your way to order a delicious-looking dessert. Don't feel guilty about it. In fact, if you don't order dessert and you really wanted dessert, we can almost guarantee that you will eventually relapse because of your self-induced deprivation. Deprivation often leads to binge eating later on. The "three bites of bliss" technique will help you avoid that.

- Go ahead and take your first bite. The first bite is indeed heavenly bliss—the most delicious thing you have ever experienced. Enjoy it. Really taste the chocolate, the nuts, the cream sauce, the cake, and the ice cream in this first bite before you swallow it. Think, "This really is worth it."

- Now you're probably thinking, "That first bite was so wonderful, I really need another one." So go ahead and take the second bite and thoroughly enjoy it.

- By now your taste buds are saturated, but for whatever reason, you want another bite! So go ahead and take that third bite. This third bite is very important for achieving satisfaction and helps you to emotionally register that you had the opportunity of selecting and eating a wonderful dessert. By letting yourself have these three bites, you prevent feelings of resentment and punishment.

- Now give the rest away, ask your waitperson to take it away, or throw the rest away. Don't worry that you've wasted it.

- Think of the power over food that you have now gained. Now you have empowered yourself with the knowledge and security that you can eat any dessert with full enjoyment, total control, and freedom from guilt.

3. Don't place any unnecessary food regulations on yourself. Avoid becoming a restricted eater, someone who is a really, really good dieter but because of self-induced restrictions eventually falls hard off his or her diet wagon. These people are the most likely to

develop all kinds of dangerous eating disorders. Do not overdedicate yourself to any rules. Keep yourself motivated toward your goal, but get there safely.

4. Remind your memory that you are eating. Focus on your meal. Turn off the TV during meals; don't read when you eat. Always sit down when you eat, even if it's only for thirty seconds. This includes eating ice cream cones at the park or zoo.

5. Make life a picnic whenever and wherever you can. Take some time to dress up your table. Eat with your best dishes and crystal. What are you saving them for? Even if you don't have time to put down a tablecloth, use an attractive cloth napkin. Buy several colors and patterns to alternate. Changing placemats also helps you remember your meal. Take a few minutes to eat your lunch outdoors and listen, feel, and experience life.

All of these food memory joggers are especially important when you are eating alone, the most common time to overeat. It is critical to follow these techniques even when you are tired after work. That may be your weakest and most vulnerable time. Start to support your food memory bank right now and you will be greatly rewarded for this investment.

# Troubleshooting

If you have followed the advice given in this book and find that you are not losing weight, ask yourself the following questions:

1. Have you noticed an improvement in the way you feel? Are you feeling less tired, more energetic, and more satisfied with the foods you eat?

- If yes, then you are on the right track to better health. Continue with the rest of the questions to determine if there may be other factors or ideas that may help with weight loss.

- If no, try decreasing the amount of high-carbohydrate foods you eat to one serving (15 grams) at each meal or snack. If this is impossible for you to do as a lifetime plan, or if you are already limiting these foods to one serving at a time, see a physician. He or she may recommend medication for insulin resistance or may order some tests to determine if there are other medical factors involved.

2. Have you increased your activity recently?

• If yes, then it is very likely that you are losing fat and increasing muscle mass, which is desirable. Since muscle is heavier than fat, you may even notice an initial increase in weight. Don't become discouraged. Remember that the more muscle mass you have, the faster your metabolism will run. You will eventually notice that you lose weight faster. Even if the scales do not show weight loss, you may have noticed that your clothes fit more loosely. It is the *fat* loss that really matters, not the weight loss.

• If no, it is time to start! Activity helps your cells to become more efficient at using carbohydrates. No weight-loss program will be successful without some kind of activity. If you have physical limitations, ask your physician or physical therapist what kind of activity would be appropriate for you. Don't believe for a second that there is nothing you can do about your situation. Remember that even small increases in activity can make a big difference.

3. Do you have cravings for high-carbohydrate foods? If yes, it is possible you are deficient in the neurotransmitters dopamine, serotonin, or histamine. Dopamine and serotonin, the regulators of appetite and cravings, are discussed in Chapter 11.

4. Are you eating enough? It is hard to imagine that eating too little may cause you not to lose weight, but this can and does happen—often! If you are not eating at least three meals each day and including at least two snacks, your body is probably in a fasting state. In this state, your body will try to conserve fat stores as much as possible. It will even burn muscle for energy instead of fat. Try eating a little more frequently—remembering to link and balance—for two weeks and see what happens. You might be fearful that you will gain weight. You may be amazed, however, that you finally begin to lose weight!

5. Are you eating too much? Even though you are limiting the high-carbohydrate foods, do you still find yourself eating large amounts of high-protein foods, dairy products, vegetables, and legumes? Do you seem to be eating constantly?

- If yes, you may be eating the same portions out of habit or you may be eating for reasons other than hunger. It is important that you eat when you are hungry and that you stop when you are satisfied for the present time. If you find that you are eating large amounts of food without any sense of fullness, perhaps you need to reevaluate your perception of how much food is enough for you. Try eating only half of the amount that you would ordinarily eat. Stop and ask yourself, "Could I stop now and be satisfied?" If the answer is yes, even though you know you could eat more and would like to eat more, you should stop. Remember that you can always eat more in another two hours.

- If you are not satisfied, take another small portion of food and repeat the process. Eat slowly, keeping in mind that none of the food you have eaten will have triggered your sense of fullness at all until *at least twenty minutes from the time you started eating.* If you eat too quickly, you can consume a large amount of food before you begin to feel satisfied.

- If you find that you are wanting to eat when you know you are not hungry, you may be eating as a response to stress or some other need, like thirst. Before you reach for something to eat, ask yourself, "What do I really need?" Be sure that your thirst is satisfied. If you then find that you are not really hungry but are in fact stressed or bored, try doing something active or relaxing for a few minutes. If you decide that you are truly hungry, try to answer the question, "What exactly am I hungry for?" before you open the cupboard. If you start out by choosing an item that will satisfy that need, you will avoid eating your way through the kitchen until that need is satisfied.

Here are some ideas that may help you eat only when you're truly hungry:

- Always take a portion of food on a plate or in a bowl and ask yourself if you are satisfied before you go back for more.

In other words, don't eat chips out of the bag or ice cream out of the container!

• Don't leave food in sight. Put it in the cupboard or, better yet, in the freezer! It won't call to you as loudly from there. Some people find that buying only a single portion of a favorite food works better than buying a whole bag and then being tempted to eat the whole thing.

• Be sure that you are not thinking of the Insulin-Resistance Diet as one that you follow when you are good, then eat whatever you want for a while when you are bad. There is no good or bad. If you eat something you feel that you should not have, get over it quickly and start right back to eating for your healthy body. Remember that eating well six days out of the week is very good. Don't dwell on the one day that you ate fast food all day!

• Don't listen to negative self-talk. If you find yourself overeating because you are convinced that you can't eat more healthfully, try telling yourself that you can do it. If you tell yourself that you are strong and successful, you will become strong and successful. You will become whatever you envision yourself to be, even if that is not how you see yourself now.

## You're on Your Way

Now that you have finished reading this book, you have developed a clearer understanding of how food really works in your body. You know how crucial controlling your insulin level is for maintaining your weight and contolling your cravings and appetite. Serious health conditions such as coronary artery disease, high blood pressure, stroke, and Type II diabetes have all been linked to insulin resistance.

Simply stated, insulin resistance is the body's way of naturally compensating for its inability to use up all the glucose made from digested carbohydrates. Rather than let dangerously high glucose levels circulate in the bloodstream, the body produces large amounts of insulin to take the glucose away. Unfortunately, this blood glucose ends up stored as fat. Strangely enough, the more insulin your body produces, the less capable your cells are of utilizing it properly. Your body becomes resistant to insulin.

We have reviewed how insulin resistance is influenced by genetics, exercise, what you eat and in what combination, and when you eat. By following our Link-and-Balance Eating Method, you can still eat the foods that you crave and love—without setting off your insulin-resistance alarm.

We know how a busy schedule sometimes makes eating at home impossible. So, in addition to the recipes that are automatically linked and balanced, we have given you practical guidelines on eating in restaurants, including fast-food restaurants.

We hope that Chapter 11 about understanding relationships with food struck a chord with you as much as it does for so many of our patients. It's amazing how often food is used to satisfy so many needs above and beyond nutrition.

If you start to lose your motivation for following this new way of eating, think of the story about Zeb and Ned. Is your tack sharp enough to get you started or to keep you going? If not, why not? Review the section "Your Values and Vision" when you need to re-commit to your goal.

We are excited for you to experience the same success that thousands of our patients have had. Thank you for letting us share with you our knowledge and experience. We look forward to hearing your success story.

# References

American College of Sports Medicine. 1978. The recommended quantity and quality of exercise for developing and maintaining fitness in healthy adults. *Medicine and Science in Sports and Exercise* 10 (3):vii–x.

Blair, S. N. 1993. *Evidence for success in exercise and weight loss and control.* Philadelphia: The American College of Physicians, 702–6.

Blundell, J. E. 1991. Pharmacological approaches to appetite suppression. *Trends in Pharmacological Science* 12:147–57.

Blundell, J. E., et al. 1993. Dietary fat and the control of energy intake: Evaluating the effects of fat on meal size and post-meal satiety. *American Journal of Clinical Nutrition* 57 (Supplement): 772s–78s.

Blundell, J. E., S. Green, and V. Burley. 1994. Carbohydrates and human appetite. *American Journal of Clinical Nutrition* 59 (Supplement):728s–34s.

Chen, I., and G. M. Reaven. 1997. Insulin resistance and atherosclerosis. *Diabetes Reviews* 5 (4):331–42.

Colaguiuri, S., and J. C. Brand Miller. 1997. The Metabolic Syndrome: From inherited survival trait to a health care problem. *Experimental and Clinical Endocrinology and Diabetes* 105 (Supplement 2):54–60.

Colby-Morley, E. 1983. Neurotransmitters and nutrition. *Journal of Orthomolecular Psychology* 12 (1):38–43.

Conte, A. A. 1993. A non-prescription alternative in weight reduction therapy. *The Bariatrician* (Summer):17–19.

DeFronzo, R. A., and E. Ferrannini. 1991. Insulin resistance: A multifaceted syndrome responsible for noninsulin dependent diabetes mellitus, obesity, hypertension, dyslipidemia, and atherosclerotic cardiovascular disease. *Diabetes Care* 14:173–94.

Dhjurandhar, N. V., and R. L. Atkinson. 1996. Development of obesity due to a human adenovirus infection. *Obesity Research* 4 (Supplement 1):24S.

Eaton, S. B., M. Shostak, and M. Konner. 1988. *The paleolithic prescription*. New York: Harper and Row Publishers.

Facchini, F. S., et al. 1992. Insulin resistance and cigarette smoking. *Lancet* (May 9) 339 (8802):1128–30.

FAO and WHO. 1998. *Carbohydrates in human nutrition*. Rome: FAO Food and Nutrition Papers, no. 66.

Fontbonne, A. 1996. Insulin resistance syndrome and cardiovascular complications of non-insulin-dependent diabetes mellitus. *Diabetes Metabolism* (October) 22 (5):305–13.

Foster-Powell, K., and J. B. Miller. 1995. International tables of glycemic index. *American Journal of Clinical Nutrition* (October) 62 (4):871S–90S.

Fu, M. M. 1995. Resistance to insulin-mediated glucose uptake and hyperinsulinemia in women who had preeclampsia during pregnancy. *American Journal of Hypertension* (July) 8 (7):768–71.

Gannon, M. C., et al. 1986. The serum insulin and plasma glucose responses to milk and fruit products in Type 2 (non-insulin-dependent) diabetic patients. *Diabetologia* 29:784–91.

Golay, A., and E. Bobbioni. 1997. The role of dietary fat in obesity. *International Journal of Obesity* 21 (Supplement 3):S2–S11.

Growden, J. 1979. Dietary influences on the synthesis of neuro-transmitters in the brain. *Nutrition Review* 37 (5):129–36.

Hausman, P., and J. B. Hurley. 1989. *The surgeon general's report on nutrition and health.* Special ed. New York: Warner Books.

Hill, A. J., and J. E. Blundell. 1991. Sensitivity of the appetite control system in obese subjects to nutritional and serotonergic challenges. *International Journal of Obesity* 14:219–33.

Hobbs, L. S. 1995. *The new diet pills.* Irvine, Calif.: Pragmatic Press.

Ivy, J. L. 1997. Role of exercise training in the prevention and treatment of insulin resistance and non-insulin dependent diabetes mellitus. *Sports Medicine* (November) 24 (5):321–36.

Karl, D. M., and M. C. Riddle. 1997. Troglitazone. *Diabetes Self-Management* (September/October):12–14.

Kelley, W. N. 1989. *Textbook of internal medicine.* Philadelphia: Lippincott.

Knowler, W. C., et al. 1978. Diabetes incidence and prevalence in Pima Indians: A nineteen-fold greater incidence than in Rochester, Minnesota. *American Journal of Epidemiology* 108: 497–504.

Kraft, J. R. 1975. Detection of diabetes mellitus in situ (occult diabetes). *Laboratory Medicine* 6:10–22.

Krezowski, P.A., et al. 1986. The effect of protein ingestion on the metabolic response to oral glucose in normal individuals. *American Journal of Clinical Nutrition* 44:847–56.

Lawton, C. L., V. J. Burley, and J. E. Blundell. 1992. Overeating of fat in obese women: Failure of high-fat intake to suppress later food intake. *International Journal of Obesity* 16 (Supplement 1):12.

Learman, L. A. 1998. Helping your patients improve their health: A primer on behavior change for obstetricians and gynecologists. *Obstetrics and Gynecology, Primary Care Update* 5 (3):130–35.

Li, E., et al. 1983. Amino acids in the regulation of food intake. *Review of Clinical Nutrition* 53:169–81.

Lyons, M. J., et al. 1982. A virally induced obesity syndrome in mice. *Science* 216:82–85.

Manson, J. E., et al. 1995. Body weight and mortality among women. *New England Journal of Medicine* 333:677–85.

McArdle, W. D., et al. 1993. *Exercise physiology: Exercise nutrition and human performance.* 4th ed. Philadelphia: Lea and Febiger.

Moore Lappé, F. 1991. *Diet for a small planet.* New York: The Ballantine Publishing Group.

National Heart, Lung, and Blood Institute. 1998. *Clinical guidelines on the identification, evaluation, and treatment of overweight and obesity in adults.* Bethesda, MD: NIH Publication, no. 98-4083, 171.

Nuttall, F. Q., and M. C. Gannon. 1991. Plasma glucose and insulin response to macronutrients in nondiabetic and NIDDM subjects. *Diabetes Care* 14:824–38.

Nuttal, F. Q., et al. 1984. Effect of protein ingestion on the glucose and insulin response to a standardized oral glucose load. *Diabetes Care* 7 (5):465–70.

Opara, J. U., and J. H. Levine. 1997. The deadly quartet—the insulin resistance syndrome. *Southern Medical Journal* (December) 90 (12):1162–68.

Panel Discussion. 1991. Factors associated with maintenance of weight loss: Prevention of relapse. *Nutrition* 7 (4):302–6.

Pavlou, K. N., et al. 1989. Exercise as an adjunct to weight loss and maintenance in moderately obese subjects. *American Journal of Clinical Nutrition* 49:1115–23.

Polivy, J. 1996. Psychological consequences of food restriction. *Journal of American Dietetics Association* 96:589–92.

Reasner, C. A. 1997. Preventing heart disease. *Diabetes Self-Management* (September/October) 14 (5):36, 38–40.

Reaven, G. M. 1995. Pathophysiology of insulin resistance in human disease. *Physiology Review* (July) 75 (3):473–86.

———. 1988. Role of insulin resistance in human disease. *Diabetes* 37:1595–1607.

Reusch, J. E. 1998. Focus on insulin resistance in Type 2 diabetes: Therapeutic implications. *Diabetes Education* (March) 24 (2):188–93.

Routtenberg, A. 1978. The reward system of the brain. *Scientific American* 239:154–65.

Saad, M. F., et al. 1988. The natural history of impaired glucose tolerance in the Pima Indians. *New England Journal of Medicine* 319:1500–1506.

Salmeron, J., et al. 1997. Dietary fiber, glycemic load, and risk of non-insulin dependent diabetes mellitus in 65,000 women. *JAMA* (February 12) 477:472–77.

Schwartz, J. M., et al. 1995. Short-term alterations in carbohydrate energy intake in humans. *Journal of Clinical Investigation* 96:2735–43.

Smith, J. R., et al. 1991. Fat and satiety: Comparison of the suppressive effect of fat and carbohydrate supplements on energy and nutrient intakes in humans. *International Journal of Obesity* 15 (Supplement):11.

Stern, M. P. 1994. The insulin resistance syndrome: The controversy is dead; long live the controversy! *Diabetologia* 37:956–58.

Stunkard, A. J., and T. A. Wadden. 1993. *Obesity: Theory and therapy.* 2nd ed. New York: Raven Press.

Trowell, H. C. 1975. Dietary-fiber hypothesis of the etiology of diabetes mellitus. *Diabetes* (August) 24 (8):762–65.

Weintraub, M. 1992. Long-term weight control: The National Heart, Lung, and Blood Institute funded multimodal intervention study. *Clinical Pharmacological Therapy* 51:581–85.

Wolever, T. M. S., et al. 1991. The glycemic index: Methodology and clinical implications. *American Journal of Clinical Nutrition* 54:846–54.

Zachweija, J. J. 1996. Exercise as treatment for obesity. *Endocrinologic Metabolism; Clinics of North America* (December) 25 (4):965–88.

Zavaoni, I., et al. 1989. Risk factors for coronary artery disease in healthy persons with hyperinsulinemia and normal glucose tolerance. *New England Journal of Medicine* 32:702–6.

Zimmet, P., et al. 1990. The epidemiology and natural history of NIDDM—Lessons from the South Pacific. *Diabetes/Metabolism Reviews* 6 (2):91–124.

# Index